William Sutherland

Sheep farming

A treatise an sheep, their management and diseases

William Sutherland

Sheep farming
A treatise an sheep, their management and diseases

ISBN/EAN: 9783742837608

Manufactured in Europe, USA, Canada, Australia, Japa

Cover: Foto ©Lupo / pixelio.de

Manufactured and distributed by brebook publishing software
(www.brebook.com)

William Sutherland

Sheep farming

"SHEEP FARMING."

A

TREATISE

ON

SHEEP,

THEIR MANAGEMENT AND DISEASES.

BY W. SUTHERLAND,
Peel Farm, Tibbermuir, N.B.

———

PRICE ONE SHILLING.

———

BERKHAMSTED:
WILLIAM COOPER & NEPHEWS,
1892.

LIST OF ILLUSTRATIONS.

INTRODUCTION.

SHEEP have been described in the "book of many meanings" as "the animals that bear wool." This definition, correct enough so far as it goes, can only be accepted as a slight instalment of the truth concerning them, since it is an unquestionable fact that amongst the members of the widespread family of ruminants there are none which are more widely diffused, or have contributed more abundantly to the necessities and comforts of mankind, from the earliest ages, than our woolly subject—the sheep.

In addition to furnishing us with wool, which the learned lexicographer seems to have considered their only merit, they are of inestimable value in supplying us with meat, suet, tallow, leather, and manure,—the latter substance proving a source of great, though indirect, advantage to mankind, by conducing in a high degree to the fertility of the soil. Sheep are now found in every part of the world where civilised man exists, in the very opposite extremes of temperature, thriving alike on the burning plains of India and on the confines of the Arctic regions.

It would be interesting were we able to determine with any degree of accuracy the period at which these valuable animals were first introduced into Britain, but unfortunately no reliable information whatever is available on that point.

There is an old saying to the effect that at one time all roads led to Rome, which was, in long past ages, the world's great seat of learning. Evidently labouring under the impression that all good gifts must of necessity have issued from that centre, some writers have asserted that sheep were unknown in this country previous to its invasion by the Romans, and have attributed their introduction to that source.

That sheep cultivation in Britain received a considerable stimulus shortly after, and directly resulting from the effects of that great historical event, is indisputable, and to the Romans is due the credit of having established, at Winchester, the first woollen manufactory of which we have any account in this country. Abundant evidence has, however, been afforded us—in the *tumuli* and cave deposits which have at different times been discovered and investigated in various districts, and which date back to eras long antecedent to the Roman invasion—that sheep existed in Britain ages upon ages before the landing of these armed marauders on her sea-girt shores, the bones of sheep having been found, mixed up with those of deer, hyenas, and even extinct animals, side by side with the rudest flint implements of early man, in those ancient deposits.

It is well known that the nature of the soil and climate exercises a powerful influence on the character of the sheep inhabiting particular situations, and that by long confinement under such fixed influences the animals in course of time acquire certain characteristics which distinguish them from others existing under different conditions, and that those characteristics are transmitted to their offspring.

It may be unhesitatingly asserted that no other country of similar extent is capable of sustaining in so great perfection such a variety of breeds, varying so much in regard to the nature of the food and climatic conditions required for their perfect welfare, as exist in Britain, and her peculiar fitness for the task is wholly due to the remarkable variety of her geological formations.

By the increasing intelligence and industry of her flockmasters, the breeds of sheep have been vastly improved within the present century. A wide field, however, still exists for experimenting in the endeavour to produce, by crossing and re-crossing existing varieties, still more profitable wool and mutton producers.

In these modern days matters are in a vastly different position from what they were fifty, ay even twenty, years ago. Improved and rapid communication has of late years made "all the world our neighbours," and the effects of foreign competition have been severely felt by the British farmer.

Stock breeders and feeders have not suffered so severely as those engaged in other branches of agriculture, and the interests of the flockmaster have not even been affected to the same extent as those engaged in cattle rearing and fee.ling, prime mutton having suffered less from foreign competition than any of the other agricultural commodities. If all tales are true, however, the competition from abroad, so far as the mutton trade is concerned, seems likely to prove much more severe in the near future than it has done in the past; it therefore behoves the sheepowner to look pointedly into every detail of his business, and, while not running rashly or hastily into "newfangled" methods of management, to be not too firmly glued to the old routine, but ready to give a fair trial to every scheme which, on being looked at from a common-sense stand-point, seems likely to result to his benefit.

One should be "ever learning," and many a useful "wrinkle" can at times be picked up in very unexpected quarters by one possessing the gift of an observant eye.

Trifles mount up—

> A *little* ill-judged parsimony here,
> A *little* unnecessary expenditure there,
> A *little* thoughtless neglect elsewhere.

Such items, when put together, form a very hurtful *whole,* and breeders and feeders alike should do "their level best" to avoid them.

SHEEP-BREEDING.

An old Scotch pedagogue, when catechising his scholars on one occasion, put to them the oft-asked query, "What is the chief end of man?" In reply he received from a precocious youngster, who had evidently studied human nature to better purpose than the contents of his "question book," the pithy and unexpected rejoinder, "Ta mak' siller."

The urchin's answer may be accepted as a clear definition of the object the sheep-breeder has in view in following his vocation, and in most cases the measure of his success is regulated by the amount of care and intelligence he exercises in the conduct of his affairs. Given careful, sensible, and systematic management, prosperity is almost assured; without these essentials, failure is just about as certain.

Whilst there are many little "odds and ends" which, when properly attended to, all contribute their quota towards ensuring success in sheep-breeding, the first and most important consideration in order to lead to the improvement— or, to put the matter in other words, to prevent the deterioration—of any flock is

CAREFUL SELECTION
of the breeding stock—both ewes and rams.

The old adage, "Like produces like," falls somewhat short of the truth. When an ill-shaped ram is put to a ewe equally defective, the probability is that the defect in the offspring will, in place of being on an equality with that of the parents, prove much more marked.

The value of a flock can, in course of time, be greatly heightened by breeding only from such animals as possess in the greatest degree the most desirable properties. All rams falling much short of the desired standard should therefore be unhesitatingly rejected ; and in whatever respect the ewes fall short of perfection (a measure rarely reached by man or sheep), care should be taken that the males selected are strong in the points in which the females are deficient. In selecting rams (and ewes also, for that matter, although the former are most important), one is never altogether safe in determining the value of the animals solely by their looks. Appearances are frequently deceptive. A very promising looking sire may be descended from very worthless ancestors, and when put to the test prove a source of serious loss to his owner by throwing stock of inferior quality. Hence the importance of

PEDIGREE,

which enables one to trace the character of the animal's "forebears." No doubt some promising-looking descendants of good stock do at times turn out unsatisfactorily, but the chances of their doing so are very much less than those whose only "character" is their own appearance.

It is, however, possible to carry respect for pedigree too far, and to persist in breeding from pedigree animals solely on account of their lineage, and without regard to their other points, is a serious error.

"In selecting rams for an ordinary breeding flock, it is well, while attaching due importance to symmetry and to good quality of flesh and fleece, to see also that the masculine features are strongly marked. The delicately formed head and neck, and placid look, which are justly admired in the ewe, and which are marks of high breeding, ought in rams to be reckoned faults, as in their case they betoken a want of size and constitutional vigour. Positive coarseness must undoubtedly be avoided; but, if this is done, better results are invariably obtained by using rams of the largest size appropriate to the particular breed, with longish heads, full crests, and a bold mien, than from neat animals of the *petit maitre* type."

IN-AND-IN BREEDING.

This subject need scarcely be touched upon. When judiciously conducted it has in some cases yielded very satisfactory results, but, if long persisted in, it exerts a very unfavourable influence on the health and vigour of the flock, and should therefore as a general rule be wholly avoided.

In every flock a thorough

"WEEDING"

should be resorted to at least once a year, and all animals of weakly constitution, or faulty in other important respects, sold off. A good class of sheep will thrive on less food, and prove more profitable in other respects, than inferior animals of the same breed—in fact, food may be said to be in great measure thrown away when expended on bad or ill-bred sheep.

INFLUENCE OF AGE OF PARENTS, ON SEX OF LAMBS.

In the early part of the present century, an interesting experiment was conducted in France, with the view of determining what influence the age of the parents had on the sex of the lambs.

At a meeting of the Agricultural Society of Severac, on 3rd July 1826, M. Charles Giron de Buzarcingues, who had previously been experimenting on the subject, and who had come to the conclusion that the sex of the lambs could be in great measure regulated at the will of the breeder, proposed that his theory should be put to a thorough test,—recommending that young rams should be put to the ewes from

which the owner desired the greater number of ewe lambs,
and that the flock should be kept on the richest and most
abundant pasture; while in regard to the ewes from which
the greater number of ram lambs were wished, he recommended that strong, vigorous, aged rams should be employed,
and that the flock should be kept on rather inferior pasture.

Two members of the Society agreed to allow their flocks
to be experimented on, and in due season the result of the
experiment was announced as follows :—

Flock for EWE lambs. Served by two rams: one 15 months, the other 2 years old.			Flock for RAM lambs. Served by two rams: one 4, the other 5 years old.		
Age of Ewes.	Sex of Lambs. M.	F.	Age of Ewes.	Sex of Lambs. M.	F.
Two years old	14	20	Two years old	7	3
Three years old	16	29	Three years old	15	14
Four years old	5	21	Four years old	33	14
	35	70		55	31
Five years old and above	18	8	Five years old and above	25	24
Total	53	84	Total......	80	55

One can scarcely accept the results of a single experiment
as altogether conclusive, still there seems a possibility that
this "wrinkle" if acted upon might be turned in some cases
to profitable account.

THE MOST DESIRABLE PROPERTIES

in any breed of sheep are hardiness of constitution, perfection
of form, early maturity and disposition to fatten, prolificness,
moderation in size, and good wool "and plenty of it."

Dealing with these virtues singly, it is manifest that

HARDINESS OF CONSTITUTION,

which is desirable in every class of sheep, in whatever quarter
they may be located, is of special importance in the case of
those reared in exposed situations, and where natural food
may at times be scarce, and artificial substitutes not easily
procurable.

PERFECTION OF FORM.

As regards this important qualification, the closer any breed of sheep approach the description given by Cully of the points desirable in a Cheviot, the nearer they are to perfection in this respect. "Head fine and small; nostrils wide and expanded; eyes prominent, bold, and daring; ears thin; collar full from breast and shoulders, but tapering gradually all the way to where the neck and head join; shoulders broad and full; mutton upon the forethigh coming quite close to the knee; legs upright with fine clean bone; breast broad and well forward; chest full and deep, not hollowed, but well filled up behind the shoulder; back and loins broad, flat, and straight; ribs rising with a fine circular arch; belly straight; quarters long and full, with mutton quite down to the hough; body covered with a thin pelt, and fine bright soft wool."

EARLY MATURITY AND DISPOSITION TO FATTEN.

These qualifications, both inducible by care in breeding and good general management are in these modern days of vital importance. Sheep possessing them yield larger profits and quicker returns to the breeder than those of slower growth. The Border Leicesters possess both these properties in a very high degree, and this has led them to be largely employed for crossing breeds deficient in these respects.

Easy corpulence has been said to be "concomitant with small bones, and also accompanied with a pliable, soft, and mellow skin."

PROLIFICNESS.

Some breeds are naturally more prolific than others; but much can be done to extend this valuable property to the less fruitful varieties by careful selection of the breeding stock, retaining only such animals as have proved themselves possessed of this important quality, and by skilful management in feeding and otherwise.

Ewes that have been reared as *pets* are almost invariably found very prolific ; and hill ewes, when removed to the more genial climate and better pasture of the lowlands, are usually found to produce a greater proportion of twin lambs than they had previously done.

MODERATION IN SIZE.

Some may be doubtful as to whether this should be regarded as a valuable point. Heavy sheep, however, generally yield coarse quality of mutton and are longer in coming to the market. It is only reasonable to suppose that they consume more food than medium-sized animals. Indeed, Sir J. B. Lawes, in reporting the results of a series of valuable experiments in sheep feeding, states that as regards the consumption of food, " Sheep of different breeds consume quantities of food in proportion to their respective weights when at an equal age, stage of feeding, &c.,—that is to say, three sheep, weighing 100 lbs. each, will consume the same quantity of food as two sheep of 150 lbs. each." And it is unquestionable that they realise considerable less per lb. when sent to the fat market than those of moderate weight.

Sheep weighing 15 or 16 lbs. per qr. when fat may be regarded as likely to yield the best return to their owner.

WOOL.

For many years back breeders in this country have devoted their attention more to improving their flocks in regard to their mutton-producing properties than in respect to the production of wool, the large importations from abroad having so seriously impaired the value of the latter commodity (reducing it in fact till, taken lb. for lb., it is of little more value than mutton) that it has been regarded as of secondary importance. Were it actually necessary to sacrifice the fleece in order to secure the greatest possible production of mutton, the fact would be sufficient to account for the inattention paid to the matter; but since there seems no reason for concluding that increased production of the one article can only be secured at the expense of the other, it may be that the subject will ere long receive more attention than has of late years been bestowed upon it.

INFLUENCE OF SOIL AND CLIMATE.

Experience has frequently and forcibly illustrated the truth of the assertion, that soil and climate exercise a powerful influence on sheep—affecting their frame, health, and power of re-production—and thus regulating, to a great extent, the bounds within which the various varieties can be bred with the greatest profit to their owner.

The rich and abundant pastures abounding in the more fertile lowland districts lead to the production of heavy, strong-boned, and fleshy animals, possessing coarse-grained flesh, deficient in flavour, and of inferior nutritive quality to the finely-grained meat yielded by the smaller-boned and lighter bodied sheep produced in hilly and mountainous districts.

CROSS-BREEDING.

Cross-breeding, accurately defined, means simply the mating of a pure bred ram of one breed with a pure bred ewe of another,—the end in view being the production of a third variety, combining the good qualities of both parents, and destitute, if possible, of the faults existing in either.

This system of breeding has done much to increase the home supply of mutton ; but in practising it great care, skill, and attention are required to ensure success, particularly when the *establishment* of a new breed is designed. Both climate and food must be suitable for the size and constitution of the animal intended to be produced ; the former more especially if a larger breed is aimed at, since softness of

constitution and tendency to disease are always increased in
proportion as additional size is acquired by crossing.

It is not actually necessary, in crossing, that both rams and
ewes should be of pure bred varieties. In many cases satisfactory results have been arrived at, in producing sheep for
ordinary butchering purposes, by employing pure bred rams
amongst cross-bred ewes. It is, however, absolutely essential
that on one side (preferably on that of the male) the animals
chosen for cross-breeding should be of pure blood. To breed
from cross-bred ewes by the aid of cross bred rams *might* in
some solitary instances lead to the production of well-pro-
portioned and valuable animals ; the chances however are,
that such a system of breeding would, in the majority of
cases, result in the yield of a race of mongrels, better fitted to
grace "Barnum's collection of curiosities" than for furnishing
a profitable return to their breeder.

BREEDING FROM LAMB RAMS

has of late years been widely practised. Looking at the
subject from a theoretical standpoint, one would be apt to
condemn the practice as likely in the long run to impair the
constitution, size, and fecundity of the flock in which the
custom was followed. Such a conclusion has, however, been
proved by the test of practice to be an erroneous one ; and
year by year the fashion gains in favour, and the demand
for ram lambs is consequently steadily increasing.

The breeders of Hampshire Downs are believed to have
been the first to attempt this system, which, having proved
satisfactory in their case, has been gradually adopted by
many owners of other varieties, even by those of black-faced
flocks.

Those who have had experience of the subject testify that
fewer barren ewes are met with in cases where ram lambs
are employed, than is usually the case when heavy shearling

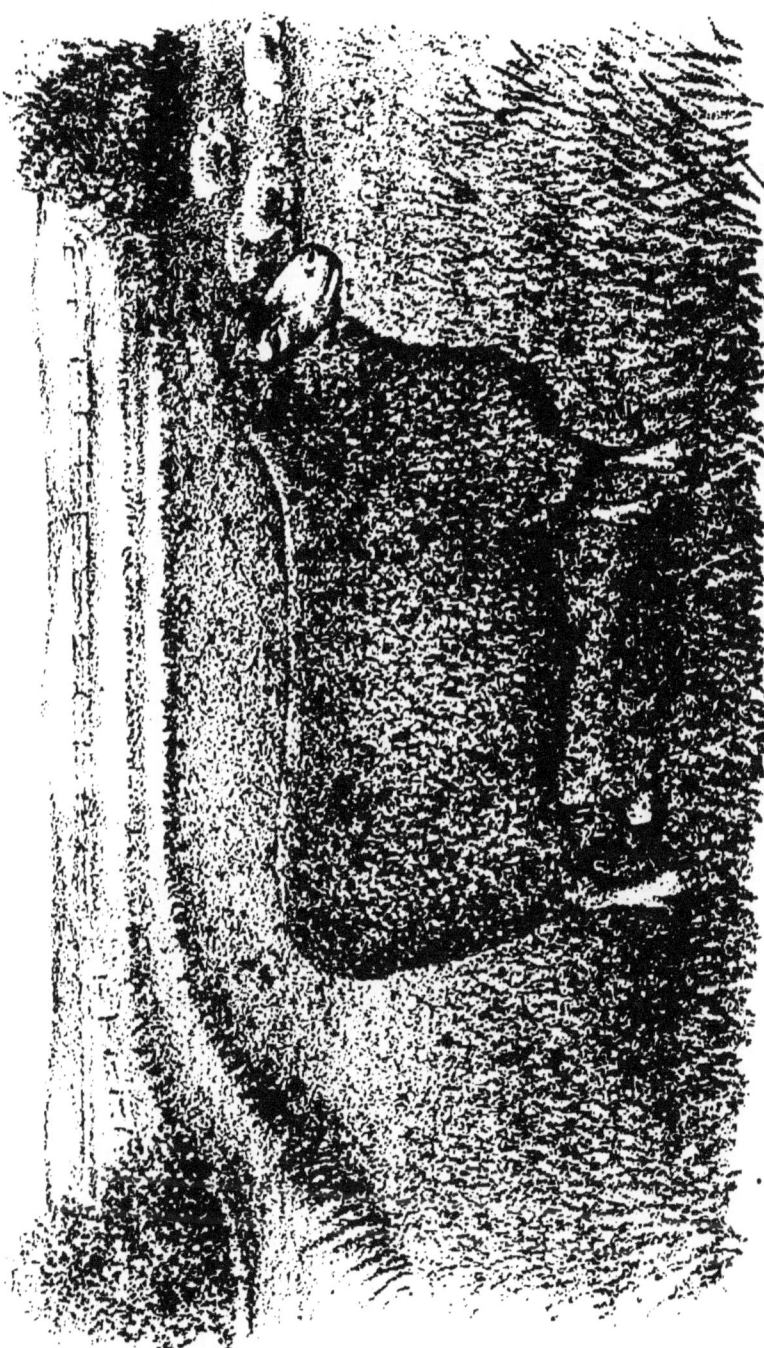

LEICESTER.

Drawn by Wm. Cooper & Nephews.

or two-shear rams are made use of. The ram lambs are also
found to "stand out" better than older tups.

The practice of

BREEDING FROM EWE LAMBS,

which is not very common, cannot be altogether favourably
spoken of. Were it possible to produce lambs from one-year-
old ewes without retarding their growth, and by treating
them in exactly the same manner in regard to feeding as
older sheep, the system would undoubtedly be very profitable.
Little penetration is, however, required to enable one to see
that this is impossible. Any attempt to carry such an unnatural system into practice, without making a liberal addition
to the diet, could scarcely fail to end disastrously ; and if
the extra expense incurred by the use of *extra nutritious*
food, and the check, which is even then put on the growth
of the animals, be taken into account—apart altogether from
the additional risk of increased mortality—the profit likely
to accrue from such breeding may be best described as "more
imaginary than real."

II.

BRITISH BREEDS OF SHEEP.

The sheep stock of Britain comprises some 25 distinct
breeds, viz.,—The Leicester, Border Leicester, Lincoln, Cotswold, Romney Marsh, Wensleydale, Devon Longwool, South
Devon, Roscommon, Southdown, Shropshire, Oxford Down,
Hampshire Down, Suffolk, Dorset, Exmoor, Dartmoor, Blackfaced, Cheviot, Half-bred, Herdwick, Lonk, Welsh, Shetland,
and Kerry breeds. Various descriptions of the breeds have
been given, *e.g,,* Lowland, Upland, and Mountain breeds, and
Long-woolled and Short-woolled, &c. ; but none of these

classifications can be made quite distinct, and so cannot be regarded as satisfactory.

THE LEICESTER

(under which term may be included the English and Border varieties, since it has been satisfactorily proved that the latter is directly descended from Bakewell's flock—the differences that now exist between the two classes being due to climatic influences, variation in management, and differences of taste amongst the breeders) may be regarded as the most important of our long-woolled breeds, arriving early at maturity, and possessing great aptitude to fatten, points which have led them to be more largely used than any other in crossing and improving other classes. When slaughtered as hoggets the mutton is of fair quality; but when aged and highly fed they do not find great favour in the eyes of the butcher, the meat being much too fat to suit the taste of his ordinary customers. The best market for such mutton is found in the large manufacturing and mining districts, the bulk of the population of which usually find it needful to make their "siller" go as far as possible, and who are therefore more particular about getting quantity than quality for their money.

THE BORDER LEICESTER

is met with over the greater portion of Scotland, and in the northern counties of England. The points of an animal of this breed have been described as follows :—

"Head of fair size, with bright lively eyes; slightly aquiline nose; muzzle full; nostril wide; face coated with clean white hair; the neck full, with strong well-developed vein; the chest broad and deep; breast well forward; shoulders broad; ribs widely arched; back broad, and firm to the touch; loins broad; quarters of good length; legs flat and clean; body well covered with a coat of fine curly wool.

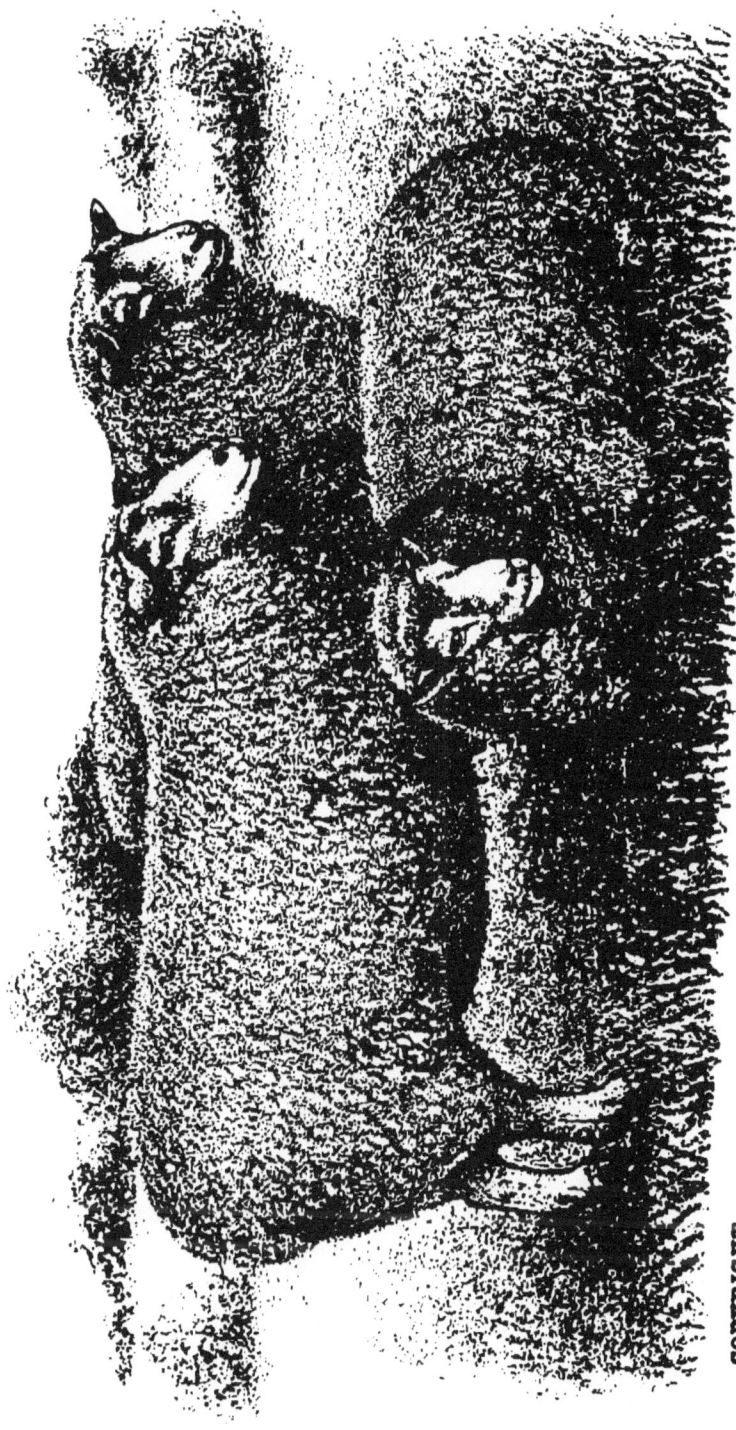

COPYRIGHT.

LINCOLN.

Drawn by Wm. Cooper & Nephews.

The animal should, in moving, carry his head well up, with ears erect, and show himself full of life and action."

ENGLISH LEICESTER.

The body of the English Leicester is smaller and more compact than that of the Border breed; the face generally of a slightly blue or dun-coloured tinge, and the head and legs covered with wool. The average fleece will weigh about 7 lbs. In many cases however this weight is considerably exceeded.

LINCOLN.

The modern Lincolns, which were obtained by crossing the old Lincoln with the new Loicester, are a valuable breed, possessing to a great extent the peculiarities of the Cotswolds and Leicesters. Tho sheep grow to an enormous size, frequently weighing 90 to 110 lbs. at twelve months old, and produce mutton of fair quality, containing a great proportion of lean meat, The ewes are hardy and prolific. The wool staple is of great length, sometimes reaching in parts of the fleece as much as 36 inches. It is bright and silky, but coarse in texture. The fleece in many instances weighs up to 12 and 14 lbs. It has of recent years been introduced for crossing purposes into Australia and New Zealand with the best results.

COTSWOLD.

The Cotswold, a native of Gloucestershire, and said to be one of the oldest classes of British sheep, is a large and hardy animal, somewhat resembling the Leicester in appearance. Its distinctive features are "a huge, long, regularly-formed body, balanced on long, clean legs ; large and noble-looking head, well woolled on the crown, long curling locks hanging down on the face ; the neck is long and thick ; back lengthy, broad, and level ; ribs well sprung ; under-line frequently somewhat irregular and defective." The Cotswolds are very prolific, and well woolled, fleece averaging 7 to 8 lbs. ; the wool is coarser on the staple than that of the Leicester. The mutton is of rather coarse quality. This breed has been much improved by a cross with the Leicester.

ROMNEY MARSH.

This breed which slightly exceeds the English Leicester in size, considerably resembles the Cheviot in appearance, and is noted as one of the closest-coated of the long-woolled varieties. The native breed was large and coarse, but a cross with the new Lincoln has produced a general improvement, and the breed is now both large and handsome. It is distinguished by a white, thick, long head, broad forehead with a tuft of wool prettily disposed upon it; long neck and carcass; good loins; thick legs and feet, and indeed large boned throughout. The wool is fine, long, closely packed and of good color, and weighs from 6½ lbs. upwards. These sheep require a good pasture and can then be run thickly upon the ground.

WENSLEYDALE.

This Yorkshire breed contains a large proportion of Leicester blood, and has been employed to a considerable extent in England for crossing blackfaced ewes. The wool is long and open·

DEVON LONGWOOL.

This variety, which contains an admixture of Cotswold and Leicester blood, is found in various parts of Devon, Cornwall, and Somersetshire, and, although of smaller make, closely resembles the Leicester in appearance.

ROSCOMMON.

The Roscommon breed are mainly confined to the province of Connaught, in the "Emerald Isle," and have, by careful management and the introduction of Leicester blood, been vastly improved since the days of Cully, who, in describing the sheep of 1800, states that they were "in almost every

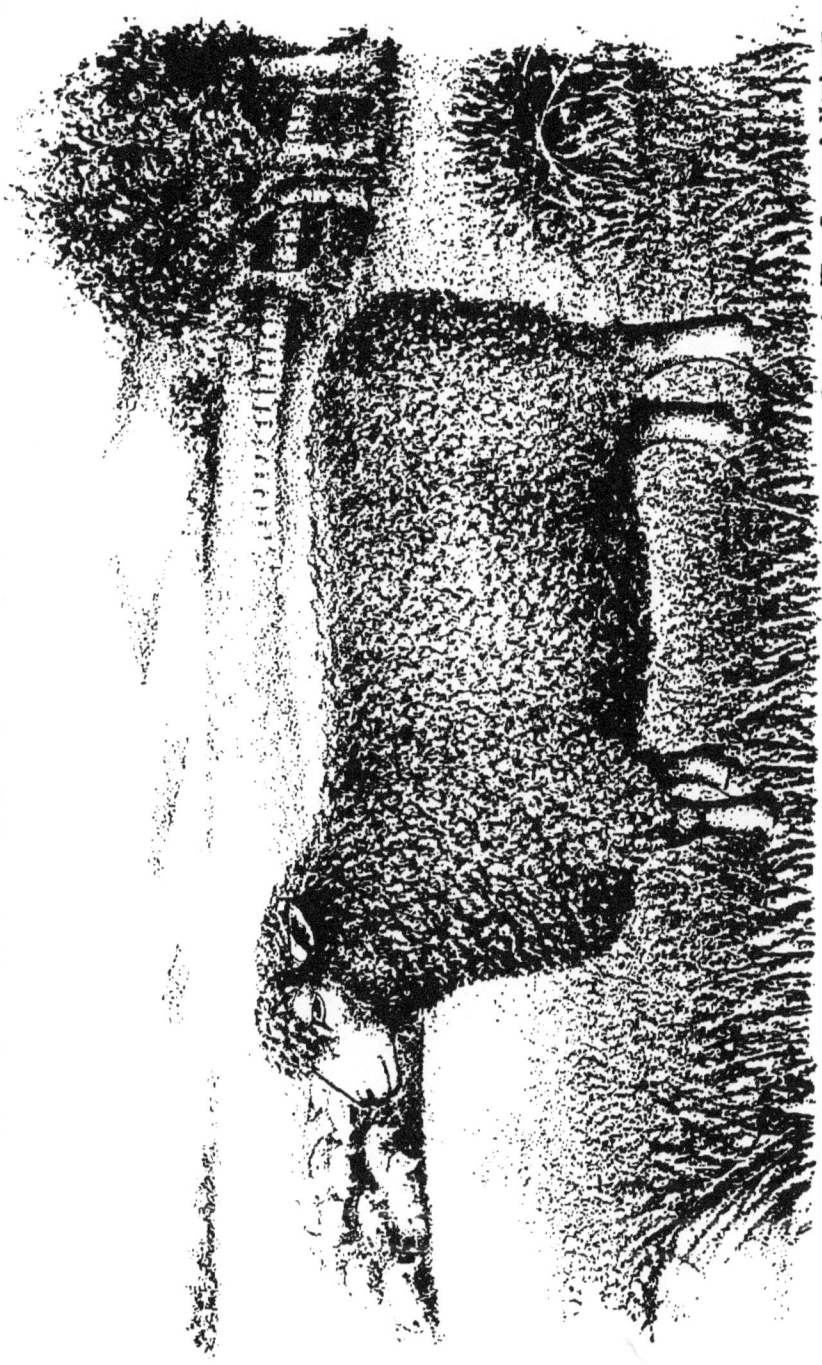

COTSWOLD.

Drawn by Wm. Cooper & Nephews.

respect the opposite of what wellbred animals should be." They are heavy mutton producers, arrive early at maturity when well fed, "kill well," and yield a heavy fleece of fine wool.

SOUTHDOWN.

No reliable information exists regarding the early history of this breed, from which all the Down varieties are descended. It has existed for generations upon the chalky soils of Sussex, and is unquestionably one of the purest and most valuable sheep in the kingdom. The modern Southdown is a perfect model of "guid gear in little bulk," being very hardy, easily kept and fattened, and yielding mutton of the finest quality. The ewes are good mothers, and usually very prolific. It has been thus described :—"The head is small and hornless, and the face brown-grey in colour, and neither too short nor too long ; the lips are thin, and the space between the eyes and nose narrow ; the under-jaw is fine and thin, while the ears are tolerably wide, and well covered with wool ; the forehead also, and the space between the ears is covered with wool ; the eyes are full and bright, but not prominent, and the orbit of the eye not too projecting ; the neck is of medium length, thin towards the head, but enlarging towards the shoulders, where it is broad and high, but straight in its whole course above and below ; the breast is wide, deep, and projecting forwards between the forelegs, indicating a good constitution and a disposition to thrive ; corresponding with this the shoulders should be on a level with the back, and not too wide above ; they should bow outwards from the top to the breast, indicating a springing rib beneath, and leaving room for it, the ribs coming out horizontally from the spine and extending far backwards, and the last rib projecting more than the others ; the back flat from the shoulders to the setting on of the tail ; the loin broad and flat, and the rump

long and broad ; the tail set on high, and nearly on a level
with the spine ; the hips wide, with the space between them
and the last rib on either side as narrow as possible, while
the ribs present a circular form like a barrel ; the belly is
straight as the back ; the legs neither too long nor too short ;
the forelegs straight from the shoulders to the foot, not
bending inwards at the knee, and standing far apart both
before and behind ; the hocks having a direction rather outwards, and the twist on the meeting of the thighs behind
being particularly full ; the bones fine, yet having no appearance of weakness, and the legs of a grey colour ; the belly
well protected with wool, and the wool coming down both
before and behind to the knee and to the hock ; the wool
short, close, curled and fine, and free from spiry projecting
fibres.   The average fleece weighs about 4 lbs."

SHROPSHIRE.

This favorite and comparatively modern breed seems capable of making itself "at home " in almost any part of the
world—flourishing in Britain, France, Germany, Canada,
United States, South America, and elsewhere—and is famed
for perfection of form, size of carcase, fine quality of mutton
(having a large proportion of lean meat to fat), arriving early
at maturity, possessing a robust constitution, and producing
good quality and weight of wool—6 to 8 lbs. per fleece. Rams
of this breed have of late years been very extensively employed for crossing purposes, and have been found very
impressive in imparting good qualities to their progeny.
"The skin should be a nice cherry colour ; the face and legs
soft black, not sooty or rusty brown, and they should be free
from all white specks, and well covered with wool."

OXFORD DOWN.

This large breed owes its origin to the crossing of Hampshire and Southdown ewes and Cotswold rams. The face is

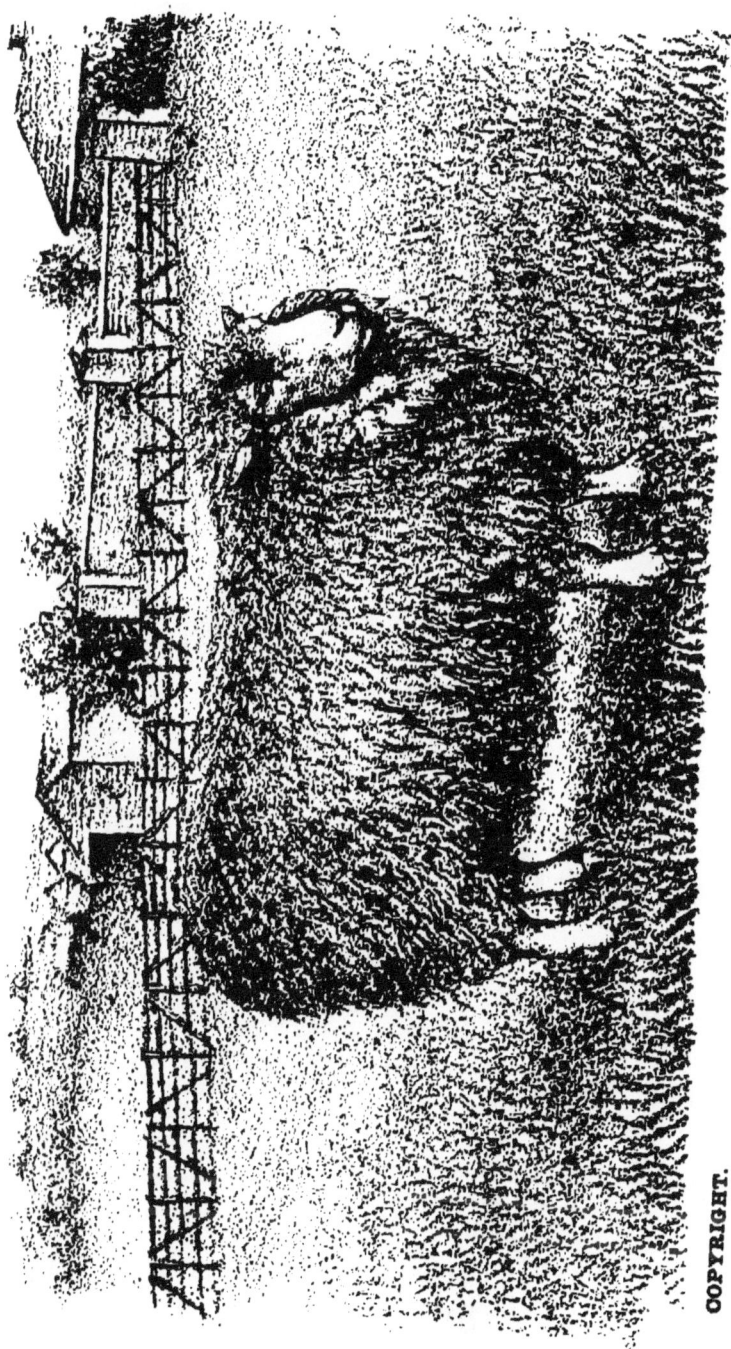

ROMNEY MARSH.

Drawn by Wm. Cooper & Nephews.

dark in colour, and the body thick and well proportioned. Oxfords are easily fattened, come early to maturity, attain heavy weights (120 to 140 lbs. at fourteen months old being nothing unusual), and produce mutton and wool of fair quality, the fleece is of fine texture, and averages 7 to 8 lbs.

HAMPSHIRE DOWN.

The modern Hampshire is the result of crossing the old breeds of Hampshire and Wiltshire ewes with Southdown rams, and may be regarded as the largest and coarsest of the Down varieties. They are not very kindly feeders, and come somewhat slowly to maturity. The wool is of fine quality, short in the staple, and averages 4 to 5 lbs. per fleece.

SUFFOLK.

This breed, formerly found very extensively in the higher lands of Norfolk, Cambridgeshire, and Suffolk, greatly resembles the Hampshire Down in appearance, but matures earlier, and excels in the production of lean mutton. It has of late been pretty generally crossed with the Southdown. Suffolks are long limbed and very active in their habits.

DORSET.

The chief peculiarity and value of this variety, one of the oldest of the English upland races, consists in the prolificness of the ewes, and in the fact that they take the ram as early as April, and are thus qualified to supply the markets with "Christmas lamb." They frequently produce two crops of lambs in the year. They are a whitefaced and horned variety, with black nose and lips, and have a tuft of wool on the forehead. Dorsets are very hardy, and easily kept, strong and active, but much wilder than the South Down. They are usually faulty in the make of their forequarters. The fleece is close, of medium quality, averaging about 5 lbs. weight.

EXMOOR.

This horned variety is chiefly found in North Devon and West Somerset. The meat is of good quality, and the wool fine and close. Average weight 4 to 5 lbs. per fleece,

BLACKFACED.

The Blackfaced, or heath-breed, as it is frequently termed, in order to distinguish it from the darkfaced forest breeds of England, is the most hardy and active of all the British varieties; capable of thriving well on scanty fare, and in severe climates which would have a ruinous effect on other breeds. Nothing definite is known as to its origin, but it is now widely diffused over the greater part of Scotland (of which it is believed to constitute about two-thirds of the entire sheep stock), and on the higher mountains of England, particularly in Westmoreland, Cumberland, and Yorkshire. The breed exists in its greatest perfection in the districts of Lanark, Ayr, and Dumfries. The wool is long, coarse, and somewhat thinly set, averaging 3½ to 5 lbs. per fleece. A Blackfaced ram should possess the following points:—"Long wool, evenly colored body with a glossy or silk appearance; legs, roots of the ears, and forehead (especially of lambs), well covered with soft fine wool; the muzzle and lips of the same light hue; the eye bright, prominent, and full of life; the muzzle long and clean, the jaw being perfectly bare of wool; the ears moderately long; the horns with two or more graceful spiral turns, springing easily from the head, inclining outwards, downwards, and forwards; the carcase long, round, and firm; the neck thick and full where it joins the shoulders; the shoulder bones well slanted; the limbs robust, the chest wide; the ribs well curved and full; wool coming well down on ribs and chest; face and legs if not entirely black should be speckled, and the hind legs well bent at the hocks, and free from black spots or "kemps." The general figure of

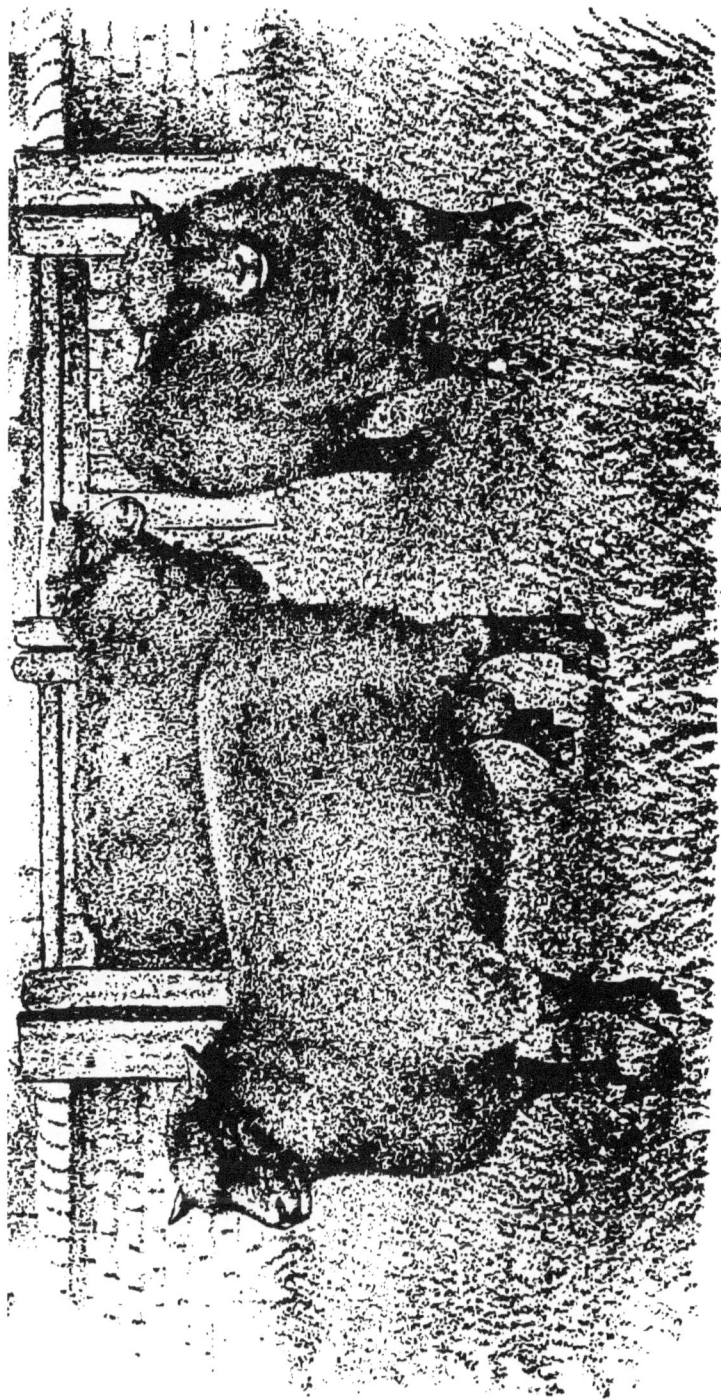

COPYRIGHT.

SOUTH DOWN.

Drawn by Wm. Cooper & Nephews.

the ewe should be the same as the tup; but the horns should be flat and "open."

Until within the last few years it was not customary to fatten off the wethers of this breed until from three to four years old. By improved management they are now brought much earlier to maturity, and it is no uncommon thing to find them sent into the fat market as hoggets. This improvement, however, has only been effected at the sacrifice, to a certain extent, of the quality of the mutton, which used to be looked upon as the finest obtainable.

CHEVIOT.

This hardy, whitefaced breed, was, as the name implies, at one time confined to the Cheviot Mountains, for the high, bare, grassy slopes of which range they are especially suitable. The superiority of their wool, which is in much request (formerly realizing as much as 2s. 6d. per lb.), led to their diffusion over large areas in Scotland, for which they were not so well adapted, at the expense of their rivals the Blackfaced breed. With the gradual depreciation in the wool value, they naturally lost favor in these regions, and in a good many cases the Scotch sheep, though less prolific, have regained the position from which they had been supplanted. The Cheviot is destitute of horns; the body is long and usually well proportioned, although there is in some flocks a tendency to lightness in the fore-quarters. The ewes are good nurses and very prolific. The mutton is superior and the fleece usually weighs from 4 to 5 lbs. When the ewes are drafted at 5 or 6 years old, they are eagerly bought by lower ground farmers, who cross them with a Border Leicester or Cotswold ram, producing the "Half-bred" sheep of the Border Counties.

HALF-BRED, OR LEICESTER-CHEVIOT CROSS.

This variety is well-known throughout Scotland and the

northern counties of England. The mutton is of good quality, containing a greater amount of lean meat than the pure Leicester. The wool, which is greatly in favour with manufacturers, is long and of fine quality, averaging 6 to 7 lbs. per fleece.

HERDWICK.

This horned breed is confined to the mountains of Westmoreland and Cumberland, in which high lying and exposed regions it is greatly appreciated on account of its hardiness of constitution. The mutton is of good quality, but the wool is coarse, and they fatten slowly. Average weight of fleece about 4 lbs.

LONK.

This variety exists mainly on the mountain ranges of Lancashire and Yorkshire, and partakes somewhat of the character of the Scotch blackfaced. The mutton is close-grained and well mixed ; the wool is short and strong on the staple, and is largely employed for blanket-making.

WELSH.

The pure bred Welsh sheep are of small size but hardy and well adapted for the mountainous districts of the principality. The quality and texture of wool varies considerably according to the pastures. On the mountain ranges it is inclined to coarseness, but when the same sheep are grazed on the lowlands the wool is of the finest quality. Great improvements have been made in this useful breed of late years. The rams are horned. The fleeces average 2 lbs. on the hills and 3 lbs. on the lowlands.

SHETLAND.

The native sheep of the Shetland Isles are of small size (seldom exceeding 10 lbs. per quarter when fat) but very hardy. During the winter season they subsist almost wholly on sea-weed, and in times of scarcity are said to be by no

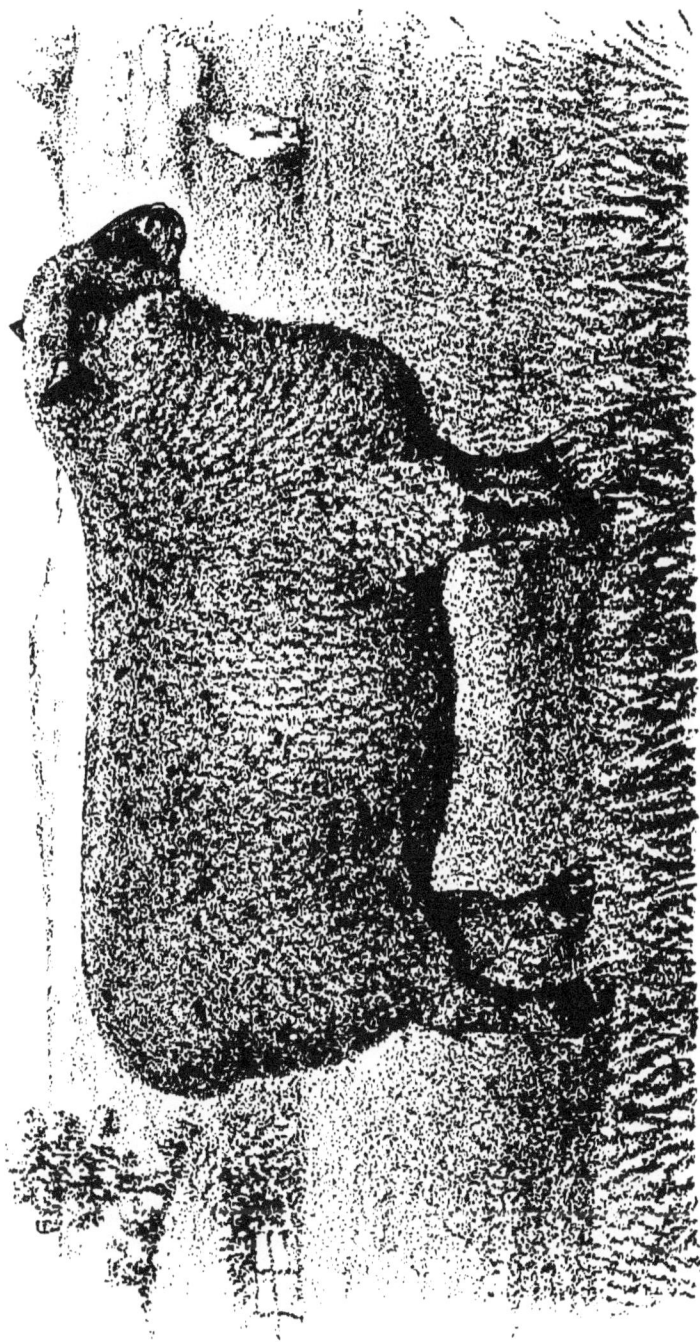

COPYRIGHT.

SHROPSHIRE.

Drawn by Wm. Cooper & Nephews.

means averse to the consumption of animal food. They are mainly esteemed on account of their fleece, which is composed of an outer coat of long hair growing through the wool, which resembles a short thick fur, thus protecting the animal from the cold while the hair throws off the wet. By a natural process the fleece becomes detached from the skin about the beginning of summer, and rises through the hair. To prevent it falling off, the sheep are gathered at the proper season and the wool pulled off by hand, the hair being thus left as a protection against cold. The fleece seldom exceeds 2 lbs. For the manufacture of hosiery goods the wool is unrivalled. In a "Description of Scotland," written at first in Latin, and "finalle translated into English by the Reverend and learned Mr. Raphael Hollinshed," it is stated in regard to the sheep stock of Shetland, that "the ewes that are to be found in these islands have for the most parte two or three lambs a piece at everie eaning." A pretty fair sample of "the good old times."

KERRY.

The old Kerry breed, widely spread at one period in the west of Ireland, is almost if not altogether extinct. Somewhat resembling, but considerably larger than the Welsh breed, these sheep are said to have been, at best, wild, coarse, and unthrifty animals, long in coming to maturity, and difficult to fatten.

In addition to the breeds already alluded to some other varieties exist; but, with two exceptions, they are so limited in numbers, and of so little more than local importance, that space will not permit reference to them.

The exceptions referred to are—(1.) The valuable class of cross-breds obtained by mating the cast ewes of the Blackfaced breed with Leicester rams. These crosses are hardy, easily fed, and great favourites with the butcher, both as lambs and hoggets, the meat being of very fine quality. The fleece is much superior to that of the blackfaced, both in weight and value. (2.) The cross between half-bred (or upland Leicester) ewes and Shropshire rams, a very superior class of sheep, the lambs being growthy, easily fattened, and greatly in favour in the fat market.

BREED STATISTICS.

From the returns recently issued by the Government it appears that the sheep stock of the United Kingdom in 1890 numbered 2,174,615. Unfortunately, however, nothing approaching accurate statistics exists to enable us to arrive at even an approximate estimate of the quota contributed by each of the breeds towards the total amount.

Compared with the figures of the previous year these returns show an increase of 546,058.

FLOCK BOOK SOCIETIES.

The necessity for " flock-books " is greater than many might be apt to imagine. Such records, in addition to preserving the character of the breed generally, add in very many cases to the value and reputation of the animals entered. American and other foreign buyers set great store on the " pedigree " of the sheep they purchase, and many of them cannot be persuaded to look at a *beast* unless the breeder can produce satisfactory references as to the lineage of his stock. Breeders of the Down varieties, which are in great demand for exportation, may almost be said to have had flock-books forced upon them.

The Shropshire, Suffolk, Oxford Down, Southdown, Hampshire, and the Wensleydale have each societies devoted to their interests, with carefully prepared registers of pedigrees; and the example set by the breeders of these classes will in all probability soon be copied by the owners of other important varieties.

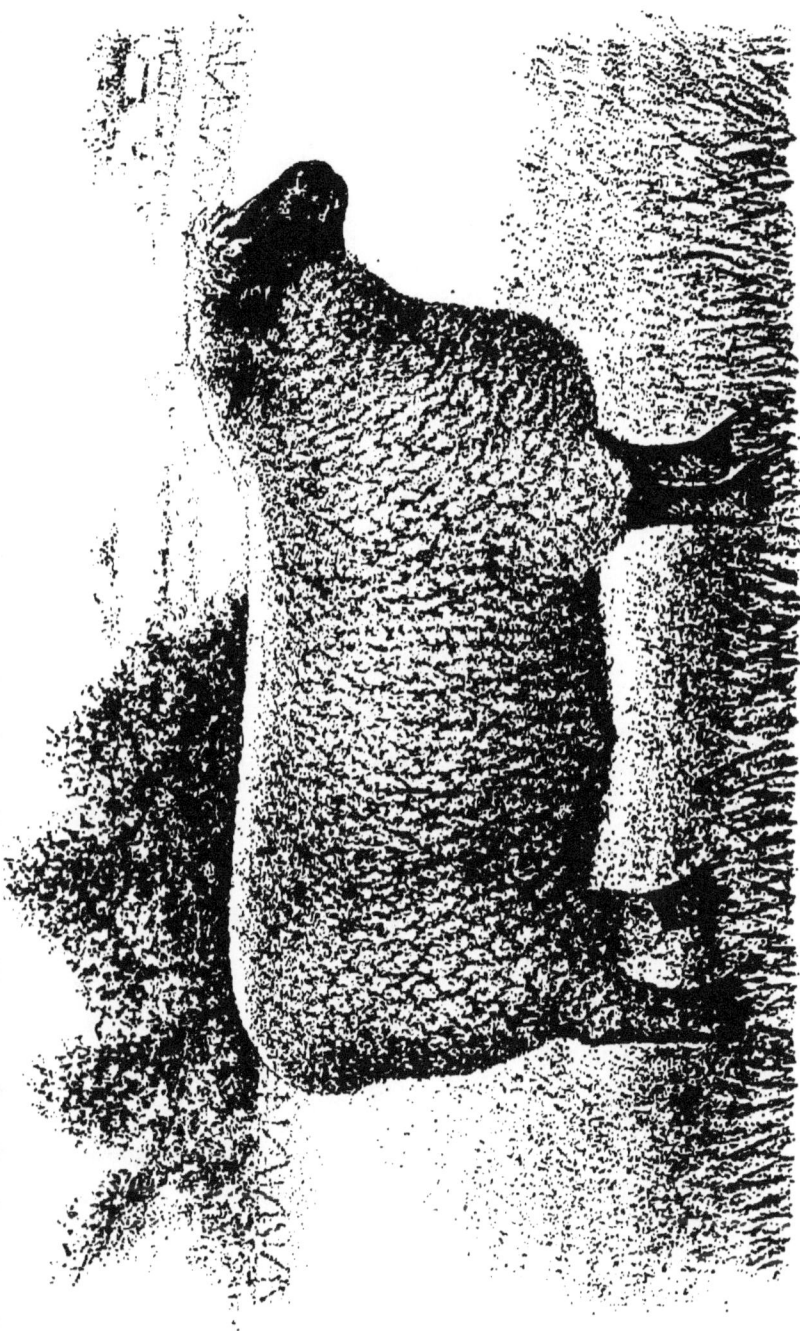

COPYRIGHT.

OXFORD DOWN.

Drawn by Wm. Cooper & Nephews.

FOREIGN BREEDS.

At the head of the foreign breeds stands the *Merino*, as to the origin of which nothing is definitely known. This breed is widely scattered, being found in various parts of Europe, and throughout North and South America, Africa and Australasia. As might be expected the Merino differs . considerably in size and appearance in the various parts of the world in which it is located. Until of late years it was cultivated more on account of its wool—which is mostly of extra quality and commands a high price—than on account of its merits as a mutton producer, in which respect it was decidedly inferior to most of the British varieties. Now, however, more attention is being bestowed upon it with the view of remedying this defect.

THE SPANISH MERINO

is described as of small size; "the males have large spiral horns, which are usually wanting in the females; the face and legs are white, though occasionally of a black or dun colour; a tuft of coarse wool grows on the forehead, and also on the cheeks; the nose and skin is of a reddish fleshy colour; there is a looseness of skin under the throat, which however unsightly to the eye of a British breeder, is esteemed a good point by Spanish shepherds as indicative of a fine fleece. The limbs are long, the sides flat, and the chest narrow; the whole structure of the animal being suggestive of an unprofitable breed so far as regards the production of mutton. The wool of this sheep excels that of every other throughout the world in fineness and quality, and in the number of its curves or serrations. From this breed the celebrated Saxony strain, and also the short necked Negretti of Austria have been derived.

RUSSIAN BREEDS.

Enormous flocks of sheep exist in this vast Empire. The .

common breed of Southern Russia has a long fat tail, is white, black, or grey, and covered with long coarse wool. This is grown for its meat, which is very toothsome. The majority of the flocks however are kept for the growth of wool. They consist chiefly of a cross between the Negretti and Rambouillét Merinos and produce very large fleeces of fine wool. In the Volga district the celebrated Astrakan breed is found, a long coarse-woolled variety mostly black. The skin of this sheep is much in request as a fur for trimming purposes.

Amongst the other foreign varieties the *Broad-tail sheep of Asia* and the *Rocky Mountain breed* are the most noteworthy. The first of these, whose caudal appendage is metamorphosed into a globular mass of delicate fat—a medium between butter and lard, and an excellent substitute for the latter—frequently weighing as much as 60 or 70 lbs., and in some instances over 100 lbs. Regarding this enormous appendage, *Buffon* states that " the tails are so long and heavy that the shepherds are obliged to fasten a small board, with wheels under them, in order to support them as the sheep walk along." In the Levant these sheep are clothed with fine wool ; in the hotter countries, such as Madagascar and the East Indies, they are clothed with hair.

The Rocky Mountain (North America) sheep is mainly remarkable for its enormous horns, which measure about 3 feet along their outer curvature from base to apex.

BRITISH SHEEP FARMING.

FOOD AND FEEDING.

Probably in no matter pertaining to the management of sheep has there been more improvement effected within the

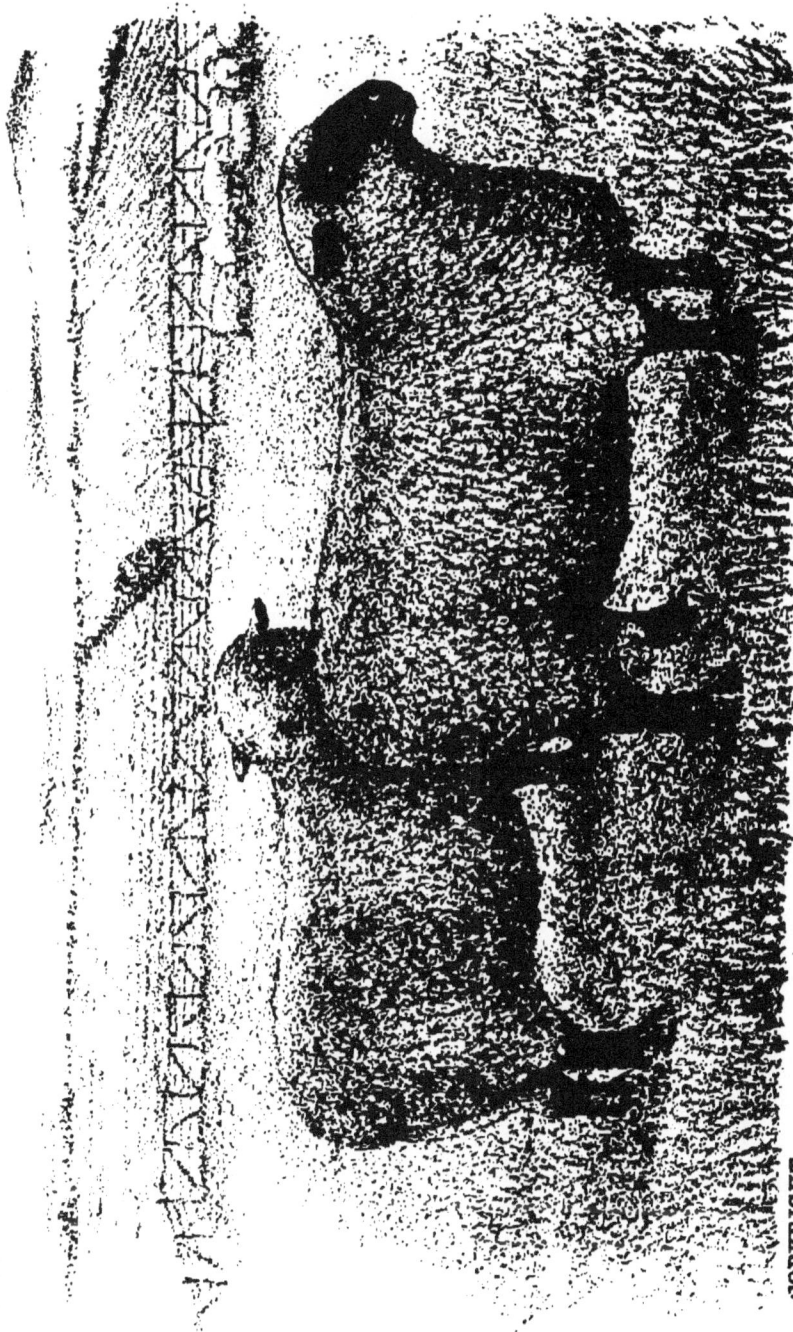

COPYRIGHT.

HAMPSHIRE DOWN.

Drawn by Wm. Cooper & Nephews.

present century than in the feeding department. In olden times the animals were left in great measure to their own devices, so far as regarded the procuring of food.

In an article which appeared in the *Farmers' Magazine* in 1807, on "The Agriculture of Ayrshire," it is stated that " The sheep are fed as God Almighty feeds the fowls of the air and the fish of the sea, upon what they can pick up themselves of nature's bounty, without the labour or assistance of man."

Nowadays the tide runs strongly in an opposite direction, and many varieties of food are supplied, the use of which for such a purpose would have been looked upon by bygone generations as sinful waste.

Although, however, great improvements have been within the present century effected as regards the food supply, there is still, in very many cases, room for further improvement. The use of imperfectly balanced food is even in these enlightened days far from being uncommon.

FEEDING SUBSTANCES.

In order to reap the greatest amount of benefit from the employment of "artificial" feeding substances, the purpose for which the animals are intended must be kept clearly in view, and the ingredients of the food adapted to that end— fattening animals being supplied with the varieties which will most rapidly lead to the accumulation of flesh and fat, and growing stock with those which are most suitable for the development of bone and muscle.

A great saving in the cost of producing mutton might ultimately be effected, were a series of experiments carefully conducted with the view of discovering what mixtures would lead to the production of the largest quantity and finest quality at the smallest expense. Many such experiments

have, it is true, been already conducted, but in several of
them some unnoticed agent has evidently influenced the
results, since the feeding substances found most profitable
in one case have not unfrequently been discovered the most
unprofitable when tested in another.

Without entering into any learned disquisition on the
elements of nutrition, fat, and general economy, a short
reference to the more common substances used as food for
sheep, and a few remarks regarding their value for that
purpose, may not come amiss.

PERMANENT PASTURE.

Grass (the nutritive value of which varies greatly according to the nature of the soil and climate) is the natural food
for sheep, and given sufficient of it of good quality all the
year round no other feeding substances would be necessary
for keeping the animals in health and condition. An unlimited or lasting supply of this valuable commodity is,
however, unfortunately unprocurable, and mainly for that
reason recourse must be had to substitutes, the most important
of which will be afterwards dealt with.

The following mixtures of Grasses and Clovers may be
recommended with Ryegrass for permanent pasture :—

NAMES OF SEEDS.	LIGHT SOILS.	MEDIUM SOILS.	HEAVY SOILS.
	lbs.	lbs.	lbs.
Dactylis glomerata (Cocksfoot)	8	6	7
Cynosurus cristatus (Crested Dogstail)	1	1	1
Festuca pratensis (Meadow Fescue)	3	6	4
Festuca ovina (Sheep's Fescue)	1	1	—
Alopecurus pratensis (Meadow Foxtail)	1½	4	3
Poa trivialis (Rough-stalked Meadow Grass)	—	1	1
Phleum pratense (Timothy or Catstail)	2	3	4
Poa nemoralis (Wood Meadow Grass)	1	¼	
Perennial Ryegrass	8	7	10
Medicago lupulina (Trefoil)	1	1	—
Trifolium hybridum (Alsike Clover)	1½	1½	2
Trifolium pratense perenne (Cowgrass Clover)	2	3	3
Trifolium repens (White Clover)	2	2	2
LBS. PER ACRE	32	37	37

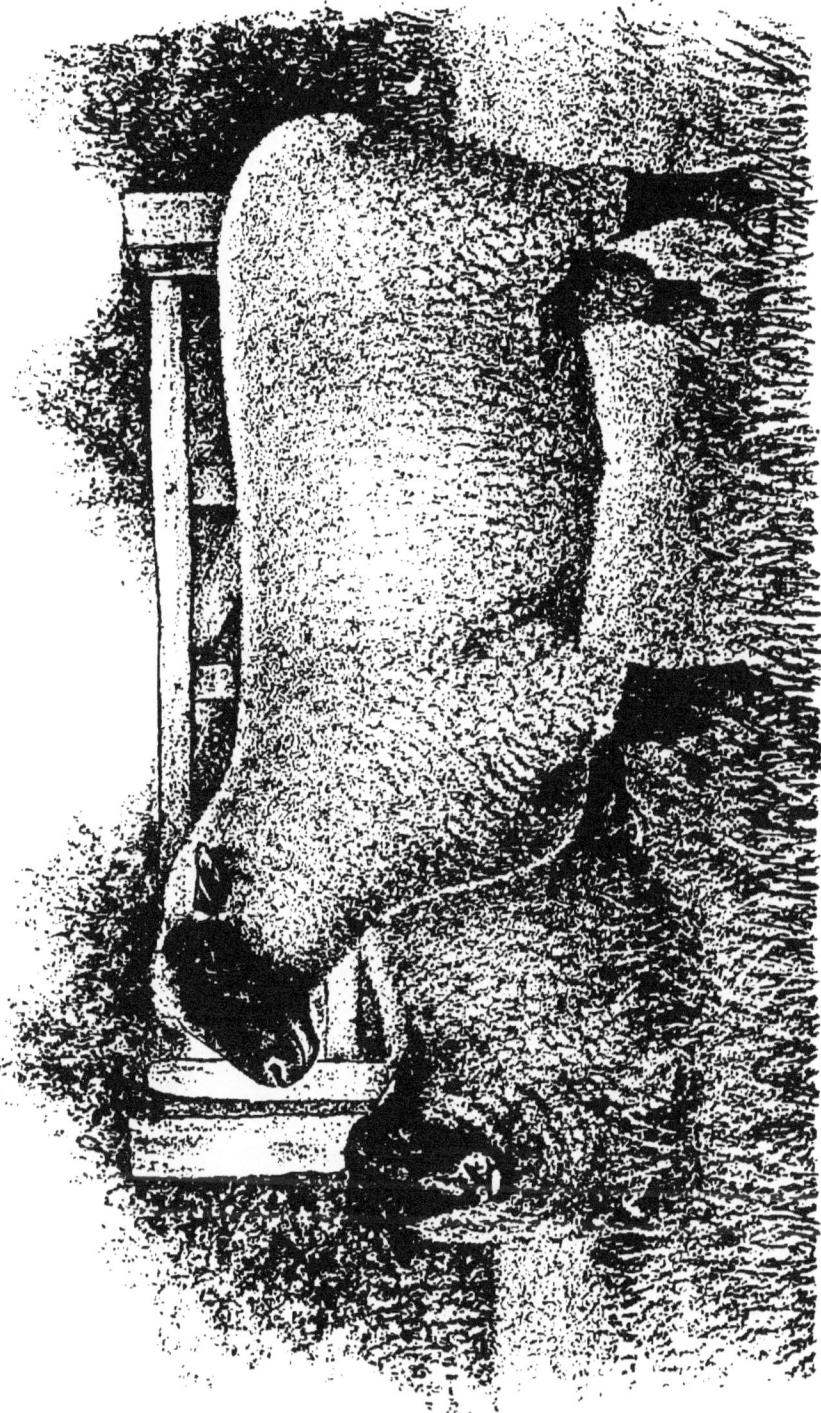

COPYRIGHT.

SUFFOLK.

Drawn by Wm. Cooper & Nephews.

Cocksfoot.—A very valuable grass; grows well on almost any soil; yields a great bulk of very nutritive feeding; should be kept closely cropped to prevent its getting tufty.

Crested Dogstail.—Very feeding close herbage, and keeps green when other grasses are dried up.

Meadow Fescue.—Very feeding, and much relished; produces heavy crop, and does well on medium and heavy soils.

Sheep's Fescue.—Slightly inferior in produce to some others, but its excellent nutritive qualities more than counterbalance the deficiency in quantity.

Meadow Foxtail.—Very early and feeding, gives big bulk, and is much relished.

Rough Stalked Meadow Grass.—Very productive.

Timothy Grass.—One of the most productive grasses known, but succeeds best on damp and heavy soils.

Wood Meadow Grass.—Produces early spring growth of fine succulent and nutritive herbage.

Perennial Ryegrass.—Suitable to all soils, and like Wood Meadow Grass is very useful for spring feeding.

Trefoil (also termed yellow clover) is an excellent fodder plant, very productive, and of rapid growth; frequently sown with sainfoin.

Alsike an extremely hardy clover, one of the very best for British pasturage.

Perennial Red or Cowgrass.—A very useful variety.

White Clover.—No pasture can be considered complete without this species. It is much in request alike for ordinary as for lawns and ornamental pasture.

OTHER FEEDING SUBSTANCES.

Sainfoin.—This plant has been cultivated in England since 1651, in which year it was introduced from France. Prior to the introduction of turnips, sainfoin was almost the mainstay of the stock-keepers on the dry and chalk soils of Wiltshire, Hampshire, and Berkshire. Even yet it is an important crop in certain of the eastern and southern counties of England. It forms a healthy and fattening food for sheep, and makes excellent hay.

Rape is extensively cultivated in various parts of England as food for sheep, and the animals fatten upon it with great rapidity. From its forcing nature it forms an admirable food for "flushing" ewes. When folded on this crop sheep should be liberally supplied with dry food to prevent "blowing."

Vetches (or tares) in their green state form a very wholesome food for sheep, and seem to possess more fattening properties than any other herbage. There are two kinds, the "Winter" and "Spring." It is advisable to sow a small area in the Autumn of the winter kind, with a quantity of winter oats, or rye added, to keep the tares off the ground when in full growth. In the Spring a succession of patches should be sown at intervals of about a month, so that a plentiful supply of this food may be at hand all the summer for folding or soiling.

Mustard is frequently sown as a forage crop for sheep, and forms a safe and healthy food. It should be stocked a week before coming into bloom to prevent it getting too "woody." For sheep feed it is usually sufficiently advanced in eight weeks from date of sowing, and from its rapid growth may be sown as a catch crop, or when turnips prove a failure.

Rye in a green state forms a valuable food for ewes and lambs in the spring months—filling the gap between the

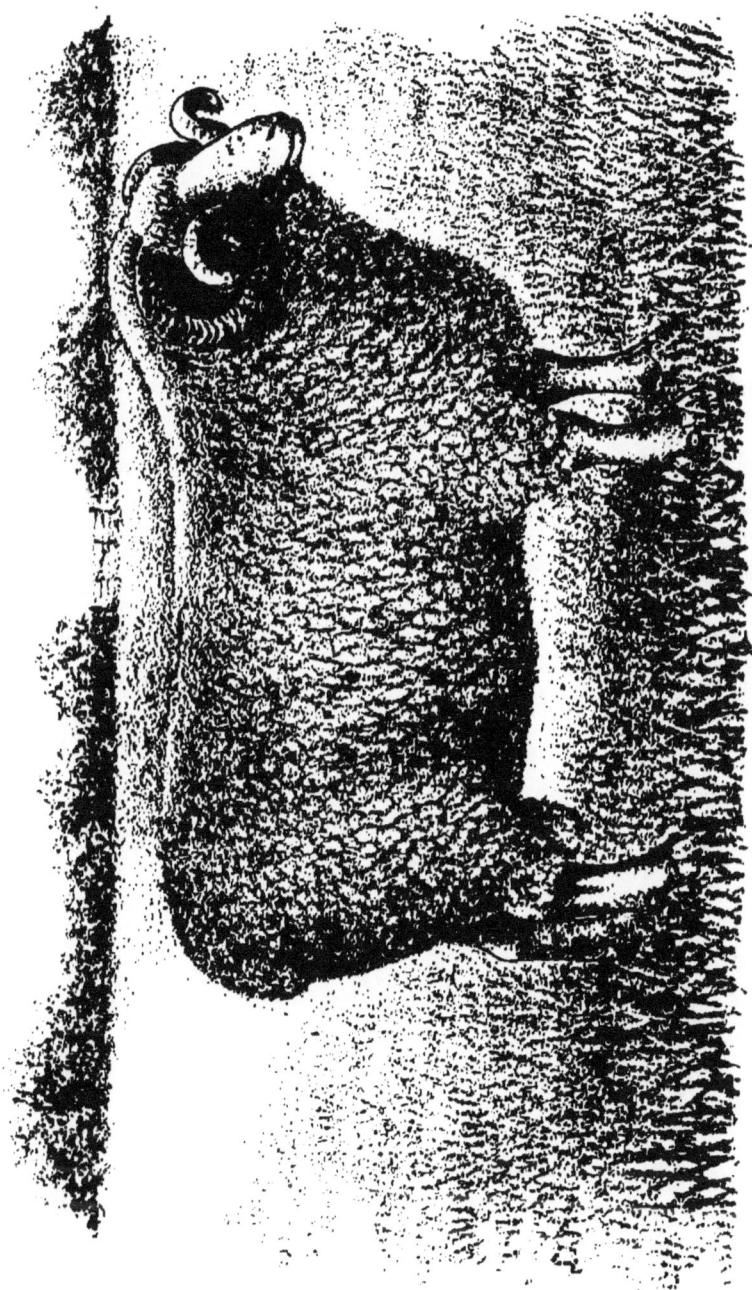

DORSET HORNED.

failure of the turnip supply and the stocking of the pastures. When allowed to get too far forward the sheep do not consume it very greedily. When intended for feeding purposes a little rape seed or a few tares are usually sown with it.

Ensilage (which is simply "the preservation of green fodder.") This method of securing the grass crop for consumption during the winter months is of immense value in wet and unfavourable seasons, when it might be impossible to convert the grass into hay without seriously impairing its feeding properties; and well-made ensilage is, as a food, decidedly superior to ill-made hay. If, however, the weather is suitable for hay-making, the preponderance of opinion is in favour of securing the crop in that shape, since the feeding properties of ensilage have not yet been proved to be equal to those of well-got hay.

Hay.—Natural grass hay, secured in good condition, forms one of the very best winter foods for sheep, and the finest quality clover hay may be said to rank next to it.

Inclement weather during the hay-making season, however, seriously damages the quality of the hay, and greatly lessens the feeding value.

Barley-straw and Oat-straw are employed to a considerable extent as fodder for sheep during the winter months, and if of good quality answer well in the case of store animals. For fattening sheep, however, the use of hay is much more profitable.

Wheat.—Average quality of wheat contains about 68 per cent. of fat and 12 per cent. of flesh formers, and at considerably over its present value may be profitably used in sheep feeding. This, and all other varieties of grain, are possibly employed to most advantage when given in mixture.

Barley, when ground into rough meal, is a valuable and largely employed feeding substance for sheep—closely resembling wheat in the proportions of flesh and fat formers.

Oats are largely used as food for growing and fattening sheep, and, owing to the large proportion of fat and flesh-forming material they contain, are admirably fitted for both purposes. They yield the most satisfactory results when bruised. If given whole, they are apt to induce inflammatory action.

Linseed Cake is a most valuable assistant to the sheep-feeder when really obtained pure. It is, however, frequently adulterated to a shameful extent, which not only lessens its feeding value, but has in some cases been the cause of serious loss to the user, on account of the nature of the impurities added to it.

Cotton Cake.—Given in moderate quantity, the decorticated variety, when procured in a soft-pressed state, is very suitable for growing sheep. The undecorticated quality is of less value and more dangerous, being apt to give rise to inflammatory attacks owing to the quantity of cotton which adheres to the seed, and its less digestible character.

Beans and Peas contain on an average about 50 per cent. of fat and 25 per cent. of flesh formers, and are better adapted for growing than fattening sheep.

Indian Corn, or maize, contains a slightly higher percentage of fat-formers, and rather less of flesh-formers, than oats. It should be ground before use.

Bran may be profitably employed in mixture with other foods, being valuable both for fattening purposes and for promoting the flow of milk in ewes rearing lambs.

Locust Beans contain fully half their weight of sugar, but are very deficient in flesh-formers, and are therefore

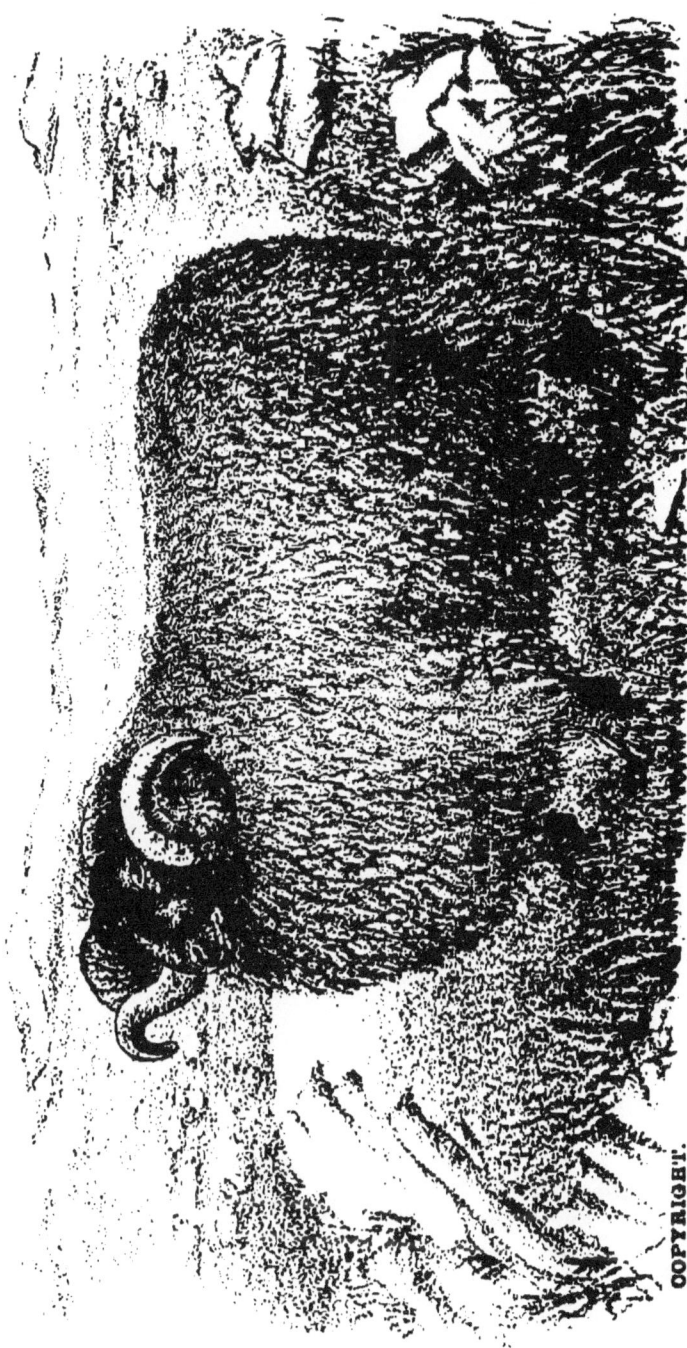

COPYRIGHT. BLACK-FACED SCOTCH. Drawn by Wm. Cooper & Nephews.

employed to most profit when given in mixture with other substances containing a high percentage of flesh-forming matter.

Brewers' grains (or Draff) tend to promote flow of milk in ewes, and when obtained in a fresh state may be usefully employed for that purpose and for mixing.

Turnips form one of the most important crops on every arable farm, and are largely employed in feeding sheep. The roots contain on an average about 90 per cent. of water. Given in reasonable quantity they are valuable for store, breeding, and fattening sheep. Fed in too great abundance they frequently lead to a heavy death-rate in the case of ewes in lamb, and in regard to fattening sheep it is usually found most profitable to limit the supply of roots, and call in the aid of other and more concentrated feeding stuffs. The *swedish* varieties are best adapted for fattening sheep. The *yellow* for store and breeding stock.

Cabbage.—In feeding properties the cabbage, taken weight for weight, closely resembles swedish turnips, but in most cases yields a much greater weight of crop per acre. Cabbages form an excellent food for sheep, and were they cultivated to a greater extent no farmer in the country need ever be in want of good keep for his flock at any season of the year.

Kale or "thousand-headed" cabbage, when well manured, yields an enormous crop of wholesome and nutritious food. This variety will pass through the hardest winter unscathed and is the best food grown for early spring feeding for ewes and lambs.

Kohl Rabi.—This plant is in reality a cabbage. It is hardier than a swede; possesses about the same feeding properties, and is best suited for dry climates and warm seasons. Sheep consume it readily and thrive well upon it.

Mangel Wurzel forms a valuable spring food for sheep, and is grown to most profit in the dry and warm climate of South England. In feeding value it is somewhat inferior to swedes, but excels them in keeping juicy and good late into spring or even into the summer.

Potatoes when at a low price can be profitably employed as food for fattening sheep, but they cannot be recommended for breeding, or for young and growing animals. Caution is necessary in commencing with them, as they are apt to disorder the stomach, and induce scour if given in too great abundance. They are best given cut, in troughs, and should, until the sheep get hardened to them, be mixed with an equal quantity of turnips.

Spiced Food.—A little spice mixed amongst the box-feeding greatly aids the laying-on of flesh, and when added to the food supplied to weakly ailing animals frequently hasten restoration to health. The excessively high prices at which these preparations are usually retailed no doubt tends to lessen the demand for them. The following ingredients are all that are required to form a high-class "spice," and the quantities mentioned about the proper proportions to keep in preparing the mixture:—

Locust-Bean meal, 56 lbs.; Indian meal, 20 lbs.; Fenugreek, 3 lbs.; Carbonate of iron, 1 lb.; Carbonate of soda, 3 lbs.; Salt, 4 lbs.

Mix the various substances thoroughly, then pass the mixture through a fine sieve, and preserve in an air-tight box. One to two ounces daily is a sufficient allowance for a sheep.

Salt.—Sheep are very fond of salt, and should have a supply of it always at their command. Its use promotes the general health and lessens the ravages of many serious disorders—liver-rot amongst them.

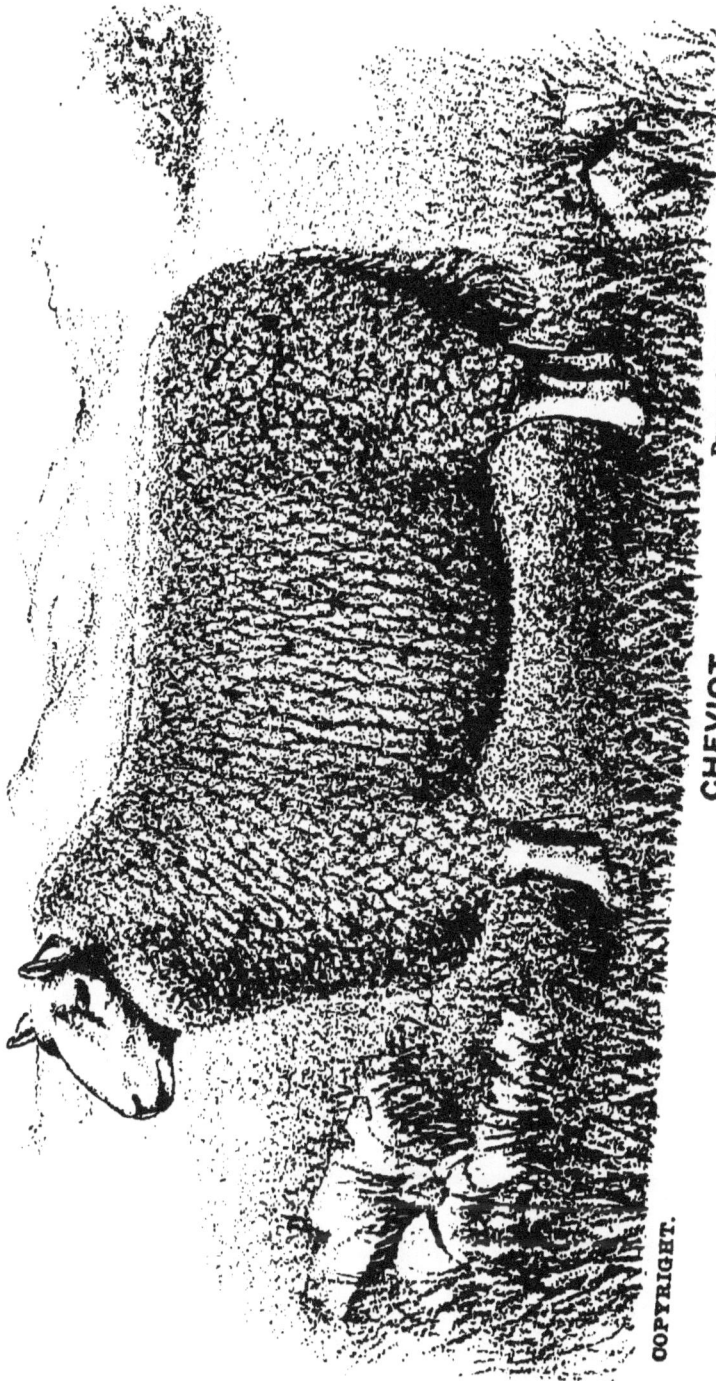

COPYRIGHT.

CHEVIOT.

Drawn by Wm. Cooper & Nephews.

It is customary in some places to give the sheep an allowance of salt amongst their food twice or thrice a week. This
system is, however, open to objection, especially in the case
of in-lamb ewes, since some of the greediest feeders may
consume more than their proper share of the food, and an
overdose of salt may cause abortion. The best method is to
keep the sheep always supplied with rock-salt, in covered
troughs reserved specially for the purpose.

WATER FOR SHEEP.

Sheep can subsist longer without water than any of our
other domesticated animals, but even in their case an abundant supply of the pure and wholesome fluid is desirable. In
the case of ewes rearing lambs, and sheep being fattened by
the aid of grain and other "artificials," access to water is of
special importance, and failure to provide it prejudicially
affects both sheep and sheep-owner—injuring the health of
the one, and curtailing the profits of the other. Free access
to water, in addition to preventing outbreaks of· certain
troubles, also enables the shepherd in many cases to detect
the presence of one fell disorder—liver-rot—at an early stage
of its existence. If sheep are observed to be very frequently
sipping water, one may rest assured that that trouble is in
existence.

METHODS OF FEEDING.

It may be said that four systems of feeding are practical—
viz., grazing, folding, house-feeding, and soiling. The business of sheep-*grazing* is mainly conducted on secondary and
inferior pasture ; the best and most feeding ground being
reserved for cattle. In order to consume the grass to the
greatest advantage close attention and skilful management
are requisite. The herbage should always, if possible, be
allowed a fair start before being stocked. Sheep bite close
to the ground, and if allowed to eat the heart out of the

plants in the early spring it frequently happens that the best
half of the grazing season is over ere the grass recovers its
vigour. Whilst, however, too early stocking is objectionable,
it is quite possible to err or the other side. If the herbage is
allowed too great a start of the sheep it is apt to become
coarse and unpalatable ; and the mischief does not end here,
since the coarsest and least valuable of the natural grasses
when left long unchecked "kill out" the less bulky but more
nutritious varieties.

"Doctors differ" as to whether it is most profitable to
stock the fields thinly and thus avoid shifting the sheep,
or to stock heavier and remove frequently from one field to
another. Provided the grass is not clipped too bare the
latter system is probably the best, since by eating "low down"
the *sole* of the pasture becomes much closer than when this
is not done, and it is also kept cleaner.

Where breeding sheep are kept, the young grass should be
reserved for the ewes and lambs ; where store and fattening
sheep only, the older pasture for the former, and the "seeds"
or young grass for the latter.

Overstocking should at all times be avoided—" whole
stocking, half profits ; half stocking, whole profits."

Folding.—This system is largely followed during the
winter and spring months ; the sheep being folded, or confined in small space, on turnips or other green crops, by
means of hurdles or nets, and a fresh "break" given them
every second or third day. The animals are found to fatten
more rapidly when kept in narrow bounds, than when they
have too great a range. In some districts it is customary to
fold the ewes and lambs on rye, or other green feeding, in
this manner during spring. In such cases the hurdles should
be arranged so that the lambs can get outside the enclosure,
and thus help themselves to the best of the food in advance
of the ewes.

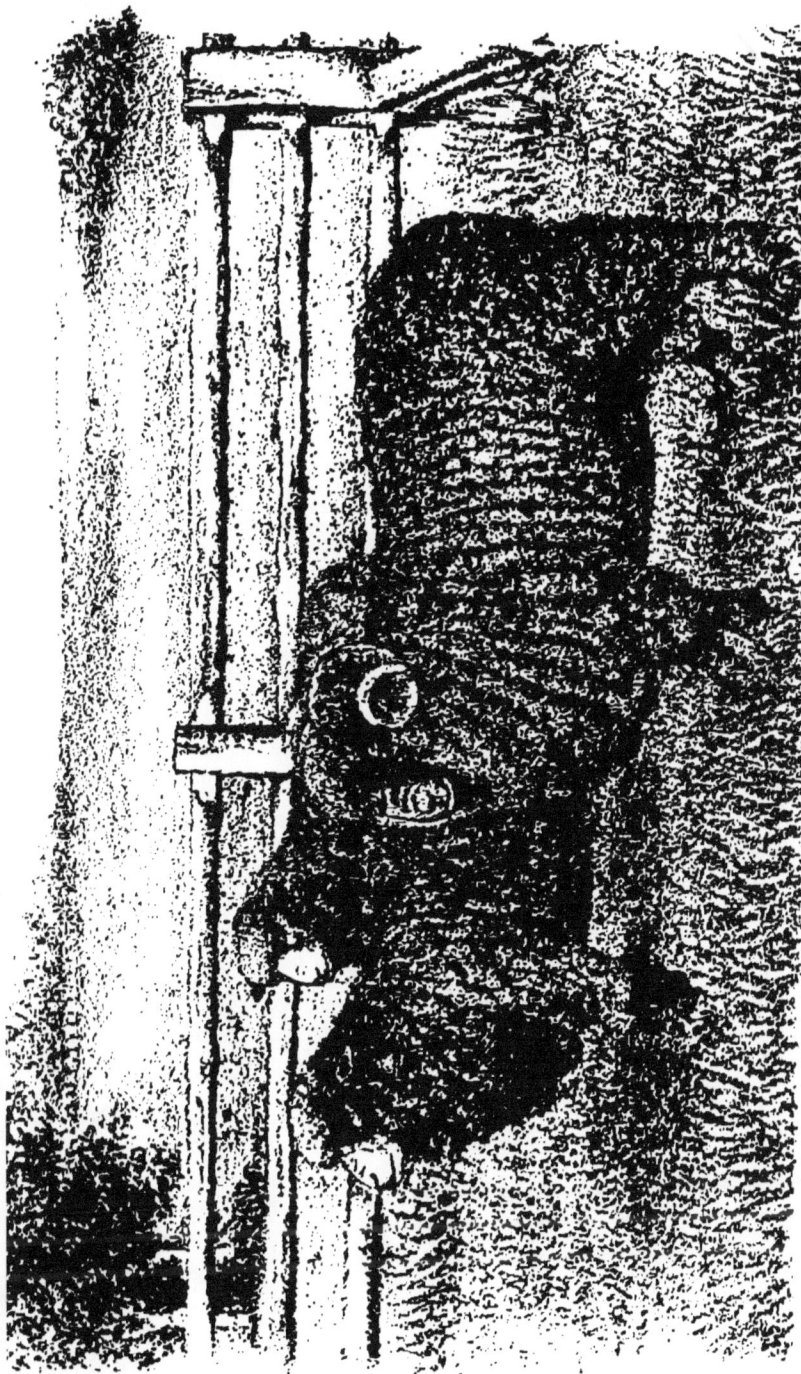

MERINO.

Drawn by Wm. Cooper & Nephews.

House Feeding.—This system is well adapted for clay land, where the sheep during wet weather would do serious injury by "poaching," and will be further referred to in another part of this treatise.

Soiling.—The term "soiling," as generally understood, refers to the consumption of green crops by stock confined in houses or open yards. When applied in the case of sheep, however, it has a wider significance. In some quarters it is customary to confine sheep on clear ground,—after potato crop or otherwise—and feed them with vetches or other substances grown on other parts of the farm ; this, and indeed the furnishing of any *extra* food to them on the pasture, is termed "soiling." On poor pastures the employment of such extras benefit both sheep and soil.

SHELTER.

In the management of sheep the provision of proper shelter for them during the prevalence of stormy weather is of the utmost importance, and possibly in no matter relating to them is more general neglect shown. In many cases no shelter whatever is provided ; in others it exists more in name than in reality. Neglect on this point undoubtedly proves a source of serious loss to the flockmaster, since exposure to furious blasts of sleety rain, or hurricanes of drifting snow, cannot fail to have a very hurtful effect on the animals, and if long continued, wastes them to a ruinous extent.

Comfortable shelter, on the other hand, is really equivalent to an increased supply of food, and tends greatly to lessen the death-rate. In every case, therefore, in which natural shelter is not available, artificial protection should be provided. The best means of affording such in varying circumstances will be alluded to further on.

APPLIANCES USED IN SHEEP-FEEDING.

The appliances necessary in sheep-feeding are not very numerous, the more important articles being hay-racks, troughs, flakes or hurdles, nets, stakes, mallet and piercer, turnip picker, turnip cutter, and cake-breaker.

Hay-racks are now generally constructed of iron, or iron and wood, and although slightly higher in first cost are cheaper in the long run than those made of wood only. Those on wheels are most convenient, as one man can easily shift them about without assistance. All racks should be provided with "economisers"— a simple and efficient one consists of a light wire railing running the whole length of the rack on each side, about 18 inches in height, standing about a foot from the rack, to which it is attached by means of cross bars bolted on the ends of the latter. By this means waste of hay is prevented, all that is pulled out and left uneaten falling between the railing and rack, in place of being trampled under foot by the sheep as it would be were this precaution not taken. Some have troughs beside the racks, which are useful for feeding with corn, &c.

Troughs are best made of wood. Those intended for feeding grain and cake should be V-shaped. For turnips and other bulky food the flat-bottomed pattern is preferable. Covered troughs are not very extensively used, being cumbersome and expensive. One or two of them are, however, useful on every farm for holding a supply of rock-salt for the sheep; to allow the brine to escape a few augur holes should be made in the bottom.

Flakes or Hurdles (usually made of larch wood) are not employed so extensively now as they were previous to the introduction of netting, in comparison with which they have three disadvantages—higher cost, greater weight, and more trouble in erecting and removing. For temporary sheep-pens, or fences seldom requiring removal, they are very useful.

Netting.—Within the last few years galvanised wire nets have to a great extent taken the place of hempen cord netting previously in common use. Where frequent shifting is necessary, cord nets are preferable to the wire ones, which are not found very durable when much handled. Cord netting, which is waterproofed with a mixture of tar and oil, is fastened to the stakes by means of ropes running along the top and bottom strands, which are hung on small hooks driven into the stakes. Wire nets are fastened by means of small staples.

Stakes should be from 4½ to 5 feet long. Those made from thinnings of larch or ash trees are most durable ; two hooks should be affixed to take the top and bottom cord of the netting.

A sharp-pointed piercer should be used, especially on hard ground, for forming the holes for the stakes, which are then driven fast by means of a hard-wood mallet.

Turnip-cutters.—The ordinary hand-cutter, a double-bladed knife, welded together in the form of an X with handle 4 feet long, is very useful for breaking turnips spread on the ground for sheep.

Cylindrical cutters, which cut the roots into finger-sized pieces, are indispensable when the sheep are being wholly fed from troughs.

In some instances cutters on this principle have been fitted on to cart-bodies, the motion being obtained from the cart wheels. As the horse moves along the turnips fall into the hopper of the cutting machine, and are cut in pieces and scattered on the ground. These turnip-cutting carts are however not likely to come into very common use, since it is only on dry ground and in very favourable weather that this system of supplying the food can be carried on without a great amount of waste.

Cake-breakers are now found on every farm where cake is employed for feeding. The cakes are placed singly in a hopper above a pair of spiked rollers, and, on motion being communicated to the machine, pass between the rollers, which can be set so as to crush to any degree of fineness required.

Turnip-pickers.—The best tool for picking the turnip shells out of the ground when the sheep consume the roots on the land where grown, is an iron fork with the prongs turned down. This should be 2 or 3 inches wide and 6 or 8 in length, fastened to a handle about 4 feet long.

BRITISH SHEEP FARMING.

SELECTION OF BREEDS.

" Circumstances alter cases," and there are many different matters which the flockmaster must take into consideration ere he can satisfactorily determine what class of sheep or what system of sheep-farming will be best suited to his particular circumstances. The character of the climate ; the nature of the soil ; the quality of the pasture, and system of cropping adhered to on arable land, have all a direct bearing on such matters. The nearness to, or distance from markets suitable for the disposal of the various descriptions of sheep should also be considered. In these days of rapid communication it may be said that " distance is no object ; " like many other sayings, however, this is only a half truth, as is manifest when one comes to consider the question of expense.

It is always best to err on the safe side, and in coming to a conclusion regarding the capabilities of his farm, it will be for the farmer's benefit to bear in mind that, in order to reap the greatest amount of profit from his flock, the qualifications of the land should in all respects be *over*, rather than under, the actual requirements of the class of stock kept upon it.

METHODS OF STOCKING.

The methods of stocking on hill-farms vary so little that no particular reference need be made to the subject at the present stage, save the mere remark that on all grazings deserving the name of "hill-farms" the ewe stock is self-maintaining.

On arable lands, however, the systems of stocking vary considerably, and in some instances the same method is not followed for two years in succession.

Regular ewe-stocks.—In many cases a regular stock of breeding ewes is kept up—the vacancies caused by the drafting or weeding of the old and defective ewes being filled up by the retention, annually, of a sufficient number of the best of the ewe-lambs. The balance of the produce, and the cast ewes, being disposed of fat, or lean, according to the capabilities of the farm.

Running ewe-stocks.—In other instances the whole produce is disposed of—the ewe-flock being maintained at a regular level, so far as numbers are concerned, by the annual purchase of the needed number of gimmers, or it may be, ewe-lambs.

Flying stocks.—Sometimes ewes, the regular casts of other flocks, are purchased in the autumn, put to the rams, and disposed of the following season in one or other of the following ways.—(1.) Just previous to lambing. (2.) With lambs at foot. (3.) Both ewes and lambs fattened, or (4.) sold separately in lean condition after weaning.

On some farms no breeding sheep are kept—store stock being brought in for the consumption of the grass during the summer, and turnips and other green crops during the winter months.

The question has been frequently put, "What system of sheep-farming is most profitable?"

The archer who has two strings to the bow is usually best off, and it may be without hesitancy asserted, that, when circumstances are suited for it, those who carry on the breeding and feeding systems combined, make, taking the average of years, the greatest profit out of their stock; and it is unquestionable that their annual returns are subject to less violent fluctations than those who are confined by necessity or choice to one system.

BREEDING RAMS FOR SALE.

The breeding of rams specially for sale for stock purposes and the letting of rams on hire for the season (a custom which now prevails to a considerable extent in various parts of England, but which has never found much favour amongst Scotch breeders, who are evidently more of the old chieftain's opinion that "each should have a boat of his own,") was first introduced in the year 1760, by Mr. R. Bakewell, of Dishley, near Loughborough, in Leicestershire.

Sharing the fate of most innovators, the encouragement bestowed upon him during the first few years was somewhat of the scantiest—indeed it is on record that he only received the miserable pittance of 17/6 for his first ram. Nothing daunted, however, he quietly persevered, and in due season perseverance brought him his well-deserved reward. Flockmasters gradually became convinced of the superiority of his sheep, and of the benefits that were likely to accrue to themselves from the use of such high-class rams in their

flocks. In the year 1784 he received £105 for a ram, and
five years afterwards an average of £420 for each of three—
whilst for part of a season's use of a famous animal, mis-
named "Two Pounder," he obtained no less than £840.

Opposition is said to be "the life of business" in many
cases it might more accurately be termed *the death of profits.*
So long as the business of ram-breeding was confined in few
hands it proved a highly profitable occupation for those
engaged in it. Of late years, however, so many have em-
barked in the trade that the profits have been reduced in too
many cases almost, if not altogether, to the vanishing point.
As a remedy for this unfortunate state of matters it has been
frequently suggested that the knife should be more freely
called into service, and none but the very best sheep retained
as rams ; and that by thus limiting the supplies prices would
be considerably heightened. Sound enough reasoning certainly—the unfortunate part of the matter is, that in this, as
in too many other matters in this wicked world, *few practice
the doctrine they preach.* "Hope springs eternal in the human
breast," and each breeder seemingly rests contented in what
proves to be the vain belief that his brother breeders will
follow the advice so freely tendered, and that consequently
he (wise man), by retaining his usual number for sale will
reap the richer harvest. ·

In some exceptional cases high prices are yet obtained ;
but, taking the whole flocks of the country into account it
is questionable, if taking one year with another, the average
for good sheep will exceed £5 per head ; whilst secondary
and unfed animals may be had at considerably less money.

Complaints are frequently heard of rams being rendered
in great measure useless by the absurd custom of overfeeding,
and in many instances there can be no doubt but that there
is only too good ground for complaint. Buyers, however,

have only themselves to blame for this hurtful practice. Just so long as sellers find that overfeeding pays them best, and no longer, will the system be continued.

A wholly unnatural method of rearing and feeding is followed by some breeders. The sheep are "housed" for the greater part of the year, and literally "stuffed" with dainties of all sorts. In addition to the usual green foods, peas, beans, oats, and other varieties of grain; cake of various sorts, locust beans, bran, boiled barley, sugar, treacle, and who knows what more are pressed into service. The animals are shorn about the beginning of January; the sheds occupied by them being afterwards kept at something approaching summer temperature, to prevent the sheep suffering from cold. When the selling season wears round these sheep make the'r appearance in the Show and Sale rings, and, as might be expected, awaken a considerable degree of admiration in the breasts of those who have not been behind the scenes. Tempted by outward appearances, purchasers are readily found, and these may reckon themselves fortunate mortals if they do not shortly afterwards discover, by dear-bought experience, the truth of the old saying, "all is not gold that glitters." When exposed to even moderately inclement weather, and although treated to *rather better* than ordinary fare, such sheep are very apt to break down in some respect, and thus betray their hot-house origin.

House-fed rams are frequently faulty on the legs; as an old shepherd once remarked "they canna walk, they only waddle."

Shelter and good feeding are undoubtedly both desirable in sheep-rearing; but when carried to extremes they become hurtful in place of beneficial.

Amongst the "fancy" prices realised at the Scotch and English Ram Sales during the Autumns of 1889 and 1890, were the following :—

Shropshires.—(1889), at the sale of Messrs. Evans, (Uffington), "Shenstone Rector," was purchased by Mr. R. P. Cooper, for £189. (1890.) The highest price realized was £210 for the ram "Windsor King" from the flock of Mr. A. E. Mansell, which was purchased for America.

Southdowns.—(1889,) at the Sale of Mr. Henry Webb's flock, at Streetly Hall, Linton, Cambs., on 3rd July, two 2-shear rams sold at £220 10s. and £199 10s. respectively. Two shearlings brought £157 10s. each ; a third £147, and a fourth £105. (1890.) From the same flock the sum of 110 guineas was this year paid at the July Sales for a shearling ram the son of "Cambridgeshire."

Hampshire.—(1889,) at Bridford Fair, on 12th August, a ram lamb from the flock of Mr. R. Moore brought £105. (1890.) Mr. More secured as much as £105 for the hire, for a month, of his champion lamb "Sanfoin."

Border Leicester.—(1889,) at the Border Union Agricultural Society's sale at Kelso, on 13th September, a shearling, the property of Messrs. Clark, Oldham-stock, sold for £108. Another belonging to the Right. Hon. Lord Polwarth, Mertoun, at £100. (1890.) The latter eclipsed his previous performance by securing £155 for a ram.

Blackfaced.—(1889), at the Perth Ram Society's 1st Sale, on 12th September, a ram bred by Mr. Fleming, Low Ploughland, sold for £90—being the highest sum ever realized up to that time for a Blackfaced sheep. (1890.) The same gentleman realized £100 for one of his celebrated rams.

Lincolns.—(1890.) Rams belonging to Messrs. J. & R. Kirkham and H. Dudding realized £105 and £99 15s. respectively.

The figures quoted above as having been realized for British bred sheep are trifling compared with those fetched in Australasia by high-class merino rams. Prices of 600 to 800 guineas are by no means uncommon, and a few years ago at the Sydney sales a Tasmanian ram brought 860 guineas.

SHEEP ON ARABLE LANDS.

SHEEP AS FERTILISERS OF THE SOIL.

Sheep are proverbially noted as the best fertilisers in existence, in so far at least as increasing the productiveness of the soil by the direct agency of live stock is concerned.

The Spaniards say that "the hoof of the sheep is golden," and attribute to it the Midas-like power of turning the land whereon it rests, to gold.

The Italians, less poetically, but more accurately, assert that "sheep are the best dung-carts," and most farmers who have had experience of the matter will readily testify to the accuracy of that assertion.

The consumption of roots and other green crops by sheep, on the land where grown, undoubtedly lays the sure foundation of a great increase in the after yield of grain and other crops, especially on light and medium soils.

The urine of sheep contains a very considerable amount of nitrogen, and furnishes ammonia on decomposition. Their manure, in addition to being more valuable, is also more beneficial than that of the other live-stock of the farm, owing to the manner in which it is distributed equally over the ground in small quantities—it is thus readily trampled into the soil by the feet of the sheep. The excrements of cattle and horses on the other hand are deposited in heaps, and soon lose a considerable amount of their value by exposure to atmospheric influences—and, in addition to this drawback, unless they are regularly and carefully spread out, one part of the ground receives overabundance of manure, (which does positive injury instead of good to the crops), whilst other portions receive nothing whatever.

The value of the manure varies according to the quality of the food supplied to the animals, and the age of the sheep has also an important bearing on the matter. In the case of full-grown sheep the elements consumed are mainly those fitted for keeping up the weight and condition of the animals. Young and growing sheep, on the other hand, extract in addition the ingredients necessary for the formation of bone and muscle, and the excrements of such animals consequently possess less manurial value.

Sheep are also valuable as

WEED DESTROYERS ;

the work of destruction being in part accomplished by the feet of the animals, but in greater measure by their cropping down many obnoxious plants—which other live-stock would pass over untouched—and thus preventing their running to seed.

***

MANAGEMENT OF BREEDING EWES.

Said a wise man of old, "Be thou diligent to know the state of thy flocks, and look well to thy herds."

In order that one may be really successful as a breeder, he must have what the late Mr. McCombie termed a "hobby" for his work, or, as an American Monthly puts it, "He must love sheep, and love to be amongst them. If a man thinks more of his own ease than of the welfare of his flock, he should leave the sheep breeding business alone." We might perhaps tone down this assertion by the addition "unless he can put some one in charge who will take a thorough interest in the proper management of matters." In most cases, however, "like master, like man," and more particularly is this so when the former is in any way remiss or careless.

FLUSHING.

The query "Does it pay to flush?" (i.e.—to supply the ewes plentifully with better food than usual for a few weeks previous to, and during the tupping season) has been answered by some in the affirmative, by others in the negative. Each breeder should, however, be best able to determine for himself as to whether the practice should, or should not, be followed in his particular circumstances. One thing is certain, if much profit is looked for from flushing, the extras given to the sheep must be, in great measure, the produce of the farm. If reliance has to be placed almost wholly on purchased feeding stuffs, it is extremely probable that the cost will swallow up the profit of the transaction.

It appears to me that flushing proves most beneficial in the case of cast ewes bought in for crossing purposes, and which it is intended to dispose of after taking one crop of lambs from them. Such ewes are generally in lean condition when purchased, and if placed on good keep, so as to put them in rapidly improving condition, they will be likely to take the ram earlier, and also to yield a better crop of lambs than they would otherwise do. In the case of regular stock ewes the flushing process is of questionable benefit; the best results (over a series of years) being most likely to be obtained by keeping the sheep as nearly as possible at a fair level of condition all the year round.

In any case in which flushing has been resorted to, care should be taken that the ewes are not allowed to fall off too much in condition afterwards, otherwise the practice may prove productive of evil instead of good.

THE TUPPING SEASON.

The duration of pregnancy in the ewe varies slightly—the

average period being from 147 to 152 days. The rams are usually placed with the ewes during the months of September and October, the earlier period being adopted in the south and the later in the north; but when early fat lambs are wanted they should be put together some weeks earlier. The number of ewes allotted to a shearling ram is usually from 50 to 60—to a ram lamb, 20 to 25.

The rams should be withdrawn from the ewes for a short period daily, and be supplied with a little extra feeding. The breast of the ram ought to be rubbed frequently with some coloring matter mixed with oil or grease, to mark the ewes when they are served, and a distinctive mark put on the ewes served by each ram in each succeeding week. By following this practice a deal of trouble is saved when the lambing season comes round, as the ewes that fall due to lamb in each successive week can then be picked out from the flock with the minimum of trouble and be put together, so that the shepherd has specially under his notice only those animals next due to lamb.

WINTER FEEDING.

No hard-and-fast rules can be laid down as to the winter feeding of in-lamb ewes—save that they should have a sufficient supply of food, and that of a suitable kind. The main endeavour should be to keep the animals in fair condition—neither too fat, nor too lean. Either extreme is objectionable; but the latter is of course most so. In the majority of cases turnips and hay constitute the bulk of the diet, a moderate allowance of box-feeding being frequently given when lambing time draws near, but of all foods given to ewes probably none is so beneficial or pays so well as an allowance of good sweet hay, and all flock-owners are strongly advised to be as generous as they can to their ewes in this way.

UDDER-LOCKING.

The old and once widely prevalent custom of removing the wool from under the tail and around the udder of the ewes, is now almost obsolete. Done, as it frequently was, before the approach of winter, the practice was a decidedly objectionable one; but when performed in moderation at the proper season—a week or two previous to lambing—less fault could be found with it; at least in the case of long-woolled ewes. If not seen to previously, every ewe should be examined shortly after lambing, and all wool likely to prevent the lambs getting freely at the teats ought to be clipped, *not pulled* away. Any suffering from scour should be carefully cleaned. If the wool about the tail is allowed to get into a filthy state, it quickly causes udder scald, and may deter the lambs from sucking, and bring about diseases in the udder.

THE LAMBING SEASON.

The old saying, "As ye sow, ye shall reap," applies with peculiar force to the flockmaster's calling. As, however, we have already dealt with the most of the preliminaries to a successful lamb-harvest, we need now only mention two other points.—(1.) That during the period of gestation the ewes should be treated with the greatest possible care—all dogging, or, at all events, all rash use of the dog—being strictly prohibited, since such is almost invariably followed by pernicious consequences, and (2), to the importance of proper shelter and lambing pens being provided for the lambing season. The shepherd should be what we may term a close-fisted individual—a veritable miser in fact, so far as his sheep are concerned; his heart set on keeping all he gets in the lamb line, out of "death's grim clutches" as long as they are under his charge. One important step towards effecting this desirable result lies in providing the animals with comfortable shelter. It is undeniable that more deaths, both of ewes and lambs, are due, directly or indirectly, to neglect in regard to this matter, than to all other causes put together. Opinions differ as to whether the erections for sheltering purposes should be of a temporary or permanent nature ; some holding to the idea that in the latter case there is greater danger of propagating disease. No doubt, if dirt and disorder rule the roast a very considerable risk is run ; but with ordinary attention to cleanliness ; thorough ventilation (but without draught), and a free use of disinfectants, any such risk is reduced to a minimum.

If no convenient buildings exist, which can be taken advantage of for sheltering purposes, the want should be met by the erection of special shelter for the sheep. This is fully dealt with under the heading of "shelter."

The erections need not necessarily be very expensive. One who is anyways "knacky," can easily run up comfortable, although possibly somewhat rough looking, shelter at wonderfully little expense. If no more substantial materials can be laid hands on, a number of flakes, or hurdles, and a quantity of well-drawn wheat, or rye straw, will fairly answer all requirements if properly put together ; perhaps no contrivance for this purpose is better than the thatched hurdle, (p. 66), for if on the one hand the ewes appear too much exposed, on the other hand all heating, which is more injurious than cold, is avoided. Sheep can stand a great amount of cold, but a hot close shed when they have heavy fleeces is most injurious.

Where many ewes are kept, and fall due to lamb early in the season, a large shed, capable of being divided into three portions, is most convenient. One end, giving access to an *uncovered enclosure*, being allotted for the unlambed ewes. The centre portion divided into pens 4 or 5 feet square, and the third division into large pens, each capable of accom-

modating a few ewes with their lambs. A separate shed,
containing a few pens, should also be erected for the accommodation of any ailing sheep—such animals should always
be strictly isolated from the healthy members of the flock,
to prevent the spread of infectious disorders.

The sheds (which should either be provided with moveable
and slightly open flooring, raised a few inches off the ground
to permit the escape of all liquid matter, or be laid with
burnt clay or ashes to a depth of 6 or 8 inches), ought to be
frequently littered with clean straw, and a weak solution of
carbolic acid, or other disinfectant, should be occasionally
sprinkled over the walls and litter, to prevent any foulness
arising.

THE LAMBING FOLD.

A week before the first of the lambs are expected, the first
served lot of ewes should be drawn out from the others, and
kept on dry ley ground, not very far removed from the fold,
during the day-time, and confined in the latter at night—the
same system being followed with the other lots successively
when they come within a week of lambing. By following
this practice the sheep get accustomed to their close quarters
before lambing commences, and, after the first night or two,
settle down contentedly as soon as they get inside. There
is thus less risk of harm being done, or loss being experienced,
than there would be were the animals only introduced to
the fold after lambing had actually commenced. The folds
should be roomy, so that the sheep do not crowd together or
become too hot, and to give the shepherd a better opportunity
of carefully noticing each animal during his visits to the fold,
which should take place frequently throughout the night.

ASSISTANCE AT LAMBING.

Once the lambs begin to make their appearance the shepherd should be constantly on the alert, but without disturbing
or unnecessarily interfering with the ewes.

Where two, or more, shepherds are kept, the work comes pretty easy, as they can take turn about in attending to the sheep. When there is only one shepherd, it is sometimes customary to hire in an assistant during the lambing season ; but most good hands prefer to see to the sheep themselves, night and day, rather than run the risk of having matters neglected, as is frequently the case when strangers are called in for a short period.

When the shepherd undertakes the two shifts himself it goes without saying that he should be assisted as much as possible during the daytime, both in the feeding of the sheep and other matters requiring attention. Untimely interference with the ewes is as much to be deprecated as the opposite fault. Experience will soon enable one to determine when assistance is, and is not, required ; and until such experience is gained one should take the advice, if he can procure it, of those who have been longer engaged at the trade than himself.

As a general rule, any ewe that does not lamb within three or four hours of the time when she first shewed symptoms of doing so will require assistance. Before affording needed help the shepherd should see that his finger-nails are short and smooth ; carefully cleanse his hands, and then lubricate them with carbolised oil (1 part of carbolic acid to 20 of sweet oil.) In rendering assistance, care and gentleness are necessary—never draw save when the ewe is pressing.

NATURAL PRESENTATIONS.

In natural presentations the lamb is always found lying upon its belly, with its head resting upon the forelegs The fore feet with the head immediately behind them are therefore presented first.

FALSE PRESENTATIONS.

False presentations are, however, by no means uncommon. In many of such cases the head only is presented, the forelegs being bent backwards. Before delivery the head should be pushed back and the legs (or at least one of them) felt for and drawn up. Should the ewe have been long in labour unnoticed, the lamb may have breathed air previous to the head being replaced. Not a moment should therefore be lost in effecting delivery, otherwise suffocation may result. In some instances only one leg is presented with the head; in such cases it is, as a rule, best to deliver the lamb in that fashion, without attempting to get forward the other leg, as the less handling the ewe gets the better.

What are termed breech presentations are often met with—in other words, the hinder part of the lamb is first presented. In such instances it is best to deliver the lamb in that position, without attempting to turn it. Should the hocks be doubled, as they frequently are, the breech must be pushed forward and the hind legs got up ere delivery can be effected, but in all these cases the experience and judgment of the shepherd must be relied on, and common sense used. In a work of this kind it is quite impossible to treat of every contingency that may arise.

It occasionally happens that some of the ewes are observed showing symptoms of lambing, but very dull and listless looking, and in no way exerting themselves. On examination in such cases the lambs will be found dead—this being at once apparent to the touch—and they must be removed by hand, a by no means pleasant, but still unavoidable task.

In all cases in which there has been much difficulty in delivery, a considerable risk—indeed, it might almost be said certainty—exists of the ewe being attacked by inflammation. With the view of warding off this disorder, a little of the carbolized oil should be passed into the womb, and two drachms of laudanum given in a little linseed gruel. When the ewe has undergone much handling, and consequently become greatly exhausted, very careful nursing will be required to aid her recovery—particularly if she is in poor condition.

In the event of any deaths occurring the shepherd should not on any account be permitted to skin the fallen sheep; especially if death has been due to inflammation, as, despite the most thorough carefulness in disinfecting himself afterwards, great danger will exist of his carrying the disorder to healthy members of the flock.

TREATMENT AFTER LAMBING.

Should the lambs seem weakly, assist them to reach the teats, and then place them with the ewe, in one of the small pens for a day or two, until they gain a little strength. Afterwards, should the weather be too severe for exposure outside, they may be drafted, a few together, into the larger pens for a time, where the lambs will have more scope for exercising their playful proclivities. There is, however, nothing worse for ewes and lambs than being cooped up for a lengthened period under cover, and they should therefore always have liberty on the pasture during the day-time, if the weather is at all favorable. It will, however, be advisable to shelter them carefully at nights till the season is pretty well advanced, in case of any sudden change taking place, and shelter of some kind should exist in the pastures. A good hedge is perhaps better than anything, but the covered hurdle or canvas shelter are most useful, and can be moved about in such a way as to ward off a great amount of wind.

Before putting many ewes with twin lambs together, each of the ewes and the lambs belonging to her should have a distinctive mark upon them; so that, in the event of anything going wrong, one can without the slightest difficulty or delay discover which belongs to which. Some might pride themselves on being able to recognise each member of their flocks without any such markings—where many sheep are kept, however, the cleverest shepherd will at times lose his reckoning, and it is therefore always best to make assurance doubly sure. It should not be necessary to say that, after the ewe has thoroughly recovered from lambing, she should be done as well as circumstances permit, for great calls will be made upon her as the lambs mature.

UNNATURAL MOTHERS.

"Can the fond ewie e'er forget
The lambkin which she bore?
Or can its plaintive cries be heard
Nor move compassion more?"

Very possibly. Gimmers, and young ewes, having twin lambs, not infrequently prove troublesome by taking to only one of the youngsters, and abusing the other. In such cases the unnatural parent should be confined in one of the small pens, and haltered in such a position as will prevent her exercising her unkindly proclivities and permit both lambs to have equal justice. A day or two of this treatment will usually suffice to convince the most stubborn offender of the error of her ways.

In the case of any aged ewes being averse to allow their lambs to suck, an examination will usually reveal the fact that sore teats are accountable for the unwillingness.

In the event of any of the ewes with twin lambs being short of milk, and others dropping single lambs about the same time having the appearance of enough and to spare, one of the twins may be removed and placed with the ewe having the single lamb. Should she seem to have any decided aversion to being burdened with the up-bringing of "ither folks bairns," why then, there's nothing for it but to administer a little of the modern cure for all obstinate-minded bipeds and quadrupeds—coercion, in the shape of a halter.

A friendly agreement will be all the more readily effected by milking the ewe and rubbing both lambs thoroughly over with the milk. By doing so the ewe is rendered unable to determine by smell which of the lambs is her own, and she usually philosophically makes the best of a bad job, by taking kindly to both.

In the event of any of the ewes having the misfortune to lose their lambs, the loss may be made so far good by placing with them lambs taken from ewes having twins. The substitutes being either rubbed over with the ewe's milk, or having the skins of the dead lambs carefully fastened on them, before being placed with their foster-mothers.

PET LAMBS.

Pets, in most cases, consist of motherless youngsters, or supernumeraries, and seem to be in general looked upon as a source of loss instead of profit. It may, however, be borne in mind that in the case of ewes having triplets it is much more profitable to remove one of the lambs and bring it up on the bottle by hand, if a more suitable foster-mother cannot be had, than to leave all three on the ewe, which would give justice neither to mother nor youngsters; and, in the case of lambs that have lost their mothers it should be borne in mind that in rearing by hand the keep of a ewe is saved. If this is taken into consideration, and matters properly managed, many farmers contend that the cost need not equal, far less exceed, the profit of the transaction.

There is no doubt a good deal of trouble connected with the upbringing of lambs in this fashion; but the individual—whatever line of life he may be in—who manages to creep along without being worried in one way or another, is unusually lucky, and if the one who has to deal with "cossets," as our American cousins call them, just accepts the bother as an unavoidable part of his daily duty, and makes the best of it, he may probably find his work just as far forward at the day's end, and with as little trouble to himself, as if the pots were not in existence.

For the first two or three weeks the lambs should have a little milk, warm from the cow, three or four times a day if the ewes have not sufficient. The exact quantity necessary will be best determined by the party giving it. The milk should, if possible, be from a cow at least a month calved, and a little dissolved sugar may, with benefit, be occasionally added to it. The best method of feeding is by means of a can fitted with an india-rubber teat at the end of a longish spout.

If milk is scarce, the lambs, once a fortnight old, may be successfully reared on one or other of the best-known calf-meals, or milk substitutes, now so commonly in use; and once they acquire an appetite for something more substantial, a small allowance of finely-ground linseed cake and bruised oats may be added to their daily fare.

SUCCOURING WEAKLY LAMBS.

Weakly lambs should never, if there seems the least likelihood of bringing them round without it, be withdrawn from their mothers, as if once removed, the ewes may not readily recognise them when they are afterwards restored, and considerable trouble may be experienced in effecting a reconciliation.

In most cases where weakness results from exposure to cold and wet, by wrapping the youngsters warmly up in woollen wraps (leaving the head exposed for the ewe to lick) and giving it a half-teaspoonful or less of gin, whisky, or brandy, in a little milk, it will quickly recover.

Animation may in many instances be restored to lambs, previously to all appearance lifeless, by keeping them immersed for a few minutes in hot water; but those brought round in this fashion require to be well looked to afterwards, as they generally turn out rather soft, and unfitted for roughing it.

The general question of rearing sheep by hand may be dismissed with the remark that they are probably more cost and trouble than they are worth, especially amongst hill sheep.

The lambing season over, the after

MANAGEMENT OF THE EWES AND LAMBS

must be regulated in accordance with the class of sheep kept, the purpose for which they are intended, and the nature of the feeding available for them.

Rearing early lambs for the fat market is now very customary in many quarters, and the lambs are frequently sold off ere the grass season has arrived.

An abundant supply of succulent green food must however be available on the farm before the rearing of early lambs can be carried on to much profit, since it is evident that without the assistance of such home-grown foods, a heavy expenditure will necessarily be incurred in the purchase of cake and other artificial feeding substances, which will of of course seriously curtail the profits.

In all cases, therefore, in which *too much* reliance has to be placed on purchased feeding stuffs, it is most profitable to arrange matters so that the lambs shall not make their appearance until there is a likelihood of a fair bite of grass being available for the ewes. A plentiful supply of turnips is so far good, but by the spring months they are frequently so dry and corky as to contain little nourishment. Unless, therefore, some other suitable home-grown food is held in reserve, a backward spring may upset all the farmer's calculations, and render a liberal supply of bought-in food indispensable if the lambs are dropped too early.

As soon as the pasture fields are ready for stocking the sheep should be placed as thinly as possible on them, or, if many are kept together, they should be frequently shifted, so that their food may be always fresh and .clean. In removing the sheep care should be taken that they are at no time suddenly transferred from short commons to a full bite of rich grass, such changes being likely to lead to outbreaks of diarrhœa.

The young seeds or first year's grass should be retained for the ewes having twin lambs, as, to give them fair play, they must be better fed than those having only one lamb each.

If the ewes are to be kept on for another season, and the lambs also retained or sold as stores, there will be little necessity for supplying them with hand-feeding if they are on fairly good pasture.

If the lambs are to be sold off fat, they should be allowed a little cake and corn ; for the first few days, until they get accustomed to the feeding, the ewes should also be allowed access to the troughs. As soon as it is seen that the lambs have acquired a taste for the food the feeding-boxes should be enclosed by hurdles, sufficient room being left beneath to admit the lambs, but not the ewes.

If it is intended to feed off the ewes also, it will generally pay to allow them a little hand-feeding. By doing so they will be got rid of early in the season when higher prices may be obtained than later on when the markets are usually filled with ewe mutton and a considerable fall in value ensues.

WEANING.

Weaning-time undoubtedly forms a red-letter period in sheep-life, since it is then that the lambs are launched out in the world on their own account,

If one can judge from the evidence afforded by eye and ear, the separation is a painful one alike to the ewes and lambs, which (if they at other times bear man's interference in their concerns with patient acquiescence,) certainly make up at this period for their past muteness by a long-continued chorus of the most piteous bleating.

Left to themselves, the ewes would suckle their offspring for nine or ten months. The gain to the lambs would, however, be more than counterbalanced by the loss in condition the ewes would sustain, and it is therefore customary to wean the lambs when about four months old.

When practicable, the ewes should be removed from the lambs, in place of the latter from the former, as the youngsters will be found to become reconciled to the loss of their mothers much more readily when left on what a Scotchman would term "*kent ground.*" When deprived of their nurses, and at the same time turned adrift on fresh pastures, they take longer to settle down contentedly. The ewes should therefore be removed out of sight and hearing of the lambs, and the latter be left confined in the fold for a few hours until the pangs of hunger begin to make themselves felt, after which they should be turned out on to the pasture ground they have previously occupied, where they may be left for a few days until they get over their bereavement.

MANAGEMENT OF LAMBS AFTER WEANING.

The after treatment of the lambs, to result profitably, must be regulated by their condition at time of weaning. The endeavour should be to keep them always improving, and if this point is neglected it simply means consumption of food without any adequate return. The stronger and higher-conditioned the lambs when weaned, the greater the necessity for treating them well afterwards.

A field of clean pasture should always be reserved for

them at this period where they can procure an abundance
of good but not over-rich food. There is nothing worse for,
or more likely to cause a heavy mortality amongst lambs,
than confining them on grass land which has been previously
heavily stocked with sheep for a lengthened period.

In many quarters it is customary to place the lambs òn
aftermath, or second crop of clover, on their removal from
the ewes. Caution is, however, needful in so doing—they
require to be gradually broken-in to such rich fare, and until
accustomed to it, should never be put on when it is wet with
dew or rain ; otherwise losses from diarrhœa, and hoove, are
almost certain to be experienced. If a field of old grass lies
adjacent to the aftermath, the best method of procedure is to
allow the lambs only an hour or two daily on the latter to
begin with, and then remove them to the old pasture. Their
period of "outing" on the more luxuriant herbage may be
daily lengthened, until, in the course of eight or ten days,
they may be confined wholly on it.

A small allowance of cake and corn tends to lessen the
risk of disease and death at this period. Access should also
be given to running water, that the lambs may freely help
themselves when they feel so disposed.

To keep sheep steadily improving in condition during the
summer season abundance of clean fresh pasture is necessary—to this end the ground must either be lightly stocked,
or frequent changes of grass must be available.

When the pasture begins to give way in the Autumn
months, sheep that are intended to be turnip-fed during the
winter season should be gradually prepared for the change
of feeding by getting a few roots daily spread and cut for
them on the leys.

MANAGEMENT OF EWES AFTER WEANING.

Care should be taken that ewes overburdened with milk

after the removal of the lambs, should have a little milk drawn from them. This is not sufficiently attended to, and bad udders are the frequent result. For a few days the ewes should be kept on a very bare pasture to check the flow of milk, and when they have fairly recovered from the separation the drafting or weeding should take place. For this purpose it is not well to trust too much to appearances or even to memory, as naturally the ewes which have done their lambs the best will be reduced in condition. A good shepherd will long since have observed and marked the faulty ewes by nipping an ear or otherwise. The drafts should be well fed until the sale. Their extra value will more than pay for the extra keep.

The reserves for breeding now often become the "scavengers" of the farm, and have to live where nothing else will. Under no circumstances, however, run your breeding ewes on wet land for it will ruin them and your flock as well.

SHEEP ON TURNIPS.

Cost of Turniping.—The cost of turniping varies greatly in accordance with the state of the crop. When the roots are in general a bulky crop throughout the country, the demand for store stock to consume them usually becomes so keen that lean sheep sell excessively dear—at rates, in fact, out of all proportion to the value of fat stock, and the price going for turnips in such seasons is consequently small. When, on the contrary, the root crop proves a partial failure, the demand for store sheep is greatly lessened, a wider margin exists between the price of lean and conditioned animals, and the letting value of the root crop is considerably greater.

CONSUMING VALUE OF TURNIPS.

The query, "What is the consuming value of turnips?" is one that has been frequently asked. This is often confused with another totally distinct question, viz: what is their "market" value. The one is a present money value, and is just what they will fetch in the market, minus the cost of getting up and transporting them; the other is a deferred value and is represented by what they will realize when converted into meat, wool, and manure for the land.

The question whether it is better to sell your turnips or keep them for growing mutton and wool depends upon a variety of considerations. If you have no sheep the matter resolves itself into a comparison of the market value with the letting value, though in the latter connection the manure produced by the sheep is an item not to be lost sight of. If you have sheep which you desire to keep, the value of the turnips will be determined by the results they will produce as against the cost of other feeding stuffs giving the same product. This must of necessity vary according to the current market price of such feeding stuffs, but it has been estimated that the equivalent of turnips in other feeding stuffs is represented by an average of about 7/6 per ton. A sheep, however, will not thrive solely on concentrated food such as oil-cake or corn, inasmuch as they are insufficient to satisfy the animal's appetite. It is always desirable, therefore, to reserve a supply of turnips in any case. As to the balance, if the market price of turnips *is less* than the cost of purchasing their equivalent in other directions it manifestly pays better to use them, as the staple article of diet. *If more,* it pays better to sell them. So much for the commercial aspect of the question.

Modes of Consuming.—In feeding sheep on the turnip crops a general practice is to "strip" the crop; one-half (more or less) being pulled and carted off for consumption by cattle, and the other half left unpulled to be eaten by the sheep on the ground where grown—two or more drills being pulled and removed, and the same number left standing in succession over the field. This system of consuming the crop is, however, open to various objections.

In the first place, the practice is a wasteful one. Even in exceptionally mild and dry winters, and on light dry land, a considerable quantity of roots are always dirtied and left uneaten, and during wet seasons and on heavy land the evil is aggravated—in many cases indeed a large proportion of the crop is destroyed or rendered unfit for food in this fashion.

Should the winter be a severe one it not unfrequently happens (as many know to their cost) that the roots are reduced by alternating frosts and freshets, to the consistency of soft soap, and rendered utterly useless so far as sheep-feeding purposes are concerned.

Apart, however, from any considerations as to waste of food, the practice should be condemned on other grounds as unnatural and unprofitable. Sheep confined on the turnip break during wet weather are of necessity subjected to a dirty diet (and to the consumption of the soil adhering to the roots many deaths must be attributed); the animals are soaked to the skin, and their beds are as miry and uncomfortable as they possibly could be—under such circumstances it is quite impossible that they can thrive satisfactorily.

Again, during the prevalance of frost the roots became so hard that, although nibbling away at them the livelong day, the poor animals often find it impossible to break off enough to satisfy their needs, and, even should they succeed in doing so, it requires little discernment to conclude that such cold frozen fare can be of but little value so far as feeding properties are concerned.

The consequences of the consumption of a large quantity of frosted roots by sheep have been likened to the effects produced on a steam-engine by the sudden in-rush of a supply of cold water. The comparison, however, is immeasurably in favour of "the iron horse"—cut off the cold current, keep up the fire, and in a few minutes he recovers his former power, with no loss, save the slight lessening of motive force for a short period. The same can scarcely be said of the sheep—the cold frozen diet tends directly to reduce condition, and it is seldom where many sheep are subjected to such treatment, but that in the case of some of them more disastrous results ensue.

To make the most of the turnip crop, it should be pulled, pitted, cut, and fed to the sheep in troughs. By adopting this system, waste of food is wholly prevented, the animals get it in a fresh and cleanly state, satisfy themselves in a short period, and have ample time afterwards to rest and be thankful; and abundance of rest, as is well enough known, is highly favourable to the laying on of condition. When the ground is dry, the sheep can, if desired, be confined and fed on the turnip land—if wet weather prevail they can be removed to the leys, where they will have the advantage of a dry bed, in place of wading to the knees, or lying in a mud-bath.

Another, and not the least important benefit gained by storing the turnips and giving them in a cut form in troughs, lies in the fact that by this system the sheep can be fed with a fixed quantity of roots daily. This cannot be done when they are confined on the turnips where grown.

That sheep may thrive to the greatest profit it is needful that they be treated in a natural manner. No class of domesticated animals require less water than our woolly friends, and it therefore follows that, when they are confined to turnips, getting as is too frequently the case, little or no dry food they are being treated unnaturally.

Turnips contain on an average about 90 per cent. of water. A three-year-old will consume at least thirty pounds weight of roots daily—*which in plain words means 27 lbs. of water*, and only 1½ lb. of fat, flesh formers, and meat-producing substances—the remaining 1½ lb. consisting of woody fibre and mineral ash.

By limiting the daily supply of roots to one-half of what the sheep would consume if supplied with an unstinted allowance, and giving the value of the other half in cake and corn, the feeder will find himself a gainer in more ways than one.

Serious losses have not unfrequently been experienced from sheep being fed almost exclusively on turnips. The winter of 1887 was specially noted in various districts in Scotland, for the heavy death-roll amongst hoggets and ewes fed in this manner. A *post-mortem* examination of some of the victims revealed the fact that the kidneys had been completely over-taxed in attempting to discharge the excessive quantity of water consumed in the roots.

When it is intended to leave the turnips unstored, and to consume them on the ground where grown, in addition to "stripping," a portion of the crop at one side of the field should be wholly removed, so that the roots may not be dirtied to the extent they would be if the sheep had no clear ground to fall back and lie on.

If the field slopes considerably, the upper portion should be first consumed ; as sheep always incline to rest on the highest and driest parts of the land.

The size of the " breaks" must be regulated by the largeness of the flock. A fresh shift should be given every second or third day at least. A plentiful allowance of good oat-straw, or hay, should always be supplied to the animals, whether box-feeding is or is not being given.

When the turnip-tops are over-luxuriant they should be

cut off, by means of a scythe, a day or two before the sheep are netted on them, to give time for them to wither.

Whilst aged sheep (provided they are not broken-mouthed,) may do fairly well on whole turnips, it is essential that, in the case of hoggets, the roots supplied after the month of January should be cut into finger-sized pieces—as at this period of the year the animals will be shedding their teeth, and are consequently unable to break the roots for themselves.

In the case of

FATTENING-SHEEP,

an allowance of box-feeding is very serviceable at this season ; the expense being amply repaid, especially on soil of secondary quality, in various ways.   The animals improve more rapidly in condition ; less grass is consumed ; a greater number of sheep can be maintained ; and the pasture is also improved by the consumption of such extra feeding on it.

Considerable difficulty is sometimes experienced in getting sheep that have not been previously accustomed to box-feeding, to take readily to it.   One method of getting over the difficulty is by confining the animals in the fold as long as may be necessary, and placing the troughs with the food beside them.   Hunger will soon tempt them to investigate the contents of the boxes, and once they get a taste of the food all trouble will be at an end.   A still better plan is to turn with flock one or two sheep that have been accustomed to box-feeding.   These will at once go to the trough, and their example will be quite sufficient to overcome the prejudice of the others.

Where many feeding sheep are kept, the most profitable method of management is to have them graded in lots, according to condition.   By this system those nearest the market can be more highly fed than the others, and are thus quickly got rid of; and as one lot is sold off the same treatment can be followed with the other lots successively.

In shifting sheep from poor to rich grass care is needful. Serious losses have occasionally been sustained by sudden removals from old leys to luxuriant young grass or aftermath. Such changes (as has been previously mentioned, in the case of lambs,) should be gradually brought about, and a dry day ought to be taken advantage of for first introducing them to such succulent feeding.

All sudden changes of condition indeed should as far as possible be avoided. Not only are they prejudicial to the sheep, but anything affecting its health injures the wool fibre, which has been called "a chart of the daily health of the sheep, whose life history is written thereon." This subject is more fully dealt with in the article on "Wool."

STORE SHEEP.

No special reference need be made to the management of store sheep. They should be treated to the best feeding available for them, so as to keep them increasing in size, if not greatly in condition.

The smallest and leanest sheep ought to be separated from the others, and fed more liberally. If this system is followed, they may be found, after the lapse of a few months, almost on an equality with the rest of the flock, which proves that a little generosity is well repaid.

SHELTER DESIRABLE.

The provision of shelter is a matter of the utmost importance in the management of fattening sheep during the winter season; since exposure to inclement weather has a very hurtful effect on the animals, always retarding their improvement in condition, and sometimes putting a stop to it altogether. Heavy loss is frequently incurred in this manner—food being consumed without any adequate return being got for it.

On most arable farms, hedges or stone-dykes exist, which may yield a certain amount of shelter during stormy weather. Failing these, a considerable measure of protection may be afforded by erecting a double row of flakes, or hurdles, and packing the space betwixt them with straw. Another economical plan is to cover a hurdle with one or two inches of straight straw, and nail strips of wood across it to keep the straw firm. In many cases it might be possible to erect, at comparatively small expense, movable shedding which would prove very beneficial to the animals during severe weather. For further remarks on this subject see page 72.

SHED OR HOUSE FEEDING.

Shed feeding has been resorted to in some cases; but except for preparing sheep for exhibition is never likely to become general. Apart from the expense of erecting suitable accommodation for the purpose, the extra attention required by the animals in such cases proves a serious obstacle to the common adoption of such a system (more especially in the case of large flocks,) even were there no other drawbacks to contend against: but it has also been found that sheep rarely do well when long confined, and unless great care is exercised foot-rot and other disorders are apt to prove troublesome. In all likelihood it will only be on stiff, or clay-land farms, that this method is at all likely to make headway. Such soil is wholly unfitted for carrying a sheep stock during the winter season; and in such instances, house-feeding—provided the animals are also allowed free access to an open yard—is perhaps the lesser of the two evils.

SHOW SHEEP.

Sheep intended for exhibition at the Royal and kindred shows are shorn and then housed as early in the season as the conditions of the competition will permit. Here for many months they are treated with the utmost liberality.

Shearing should always precede the housing, otherwise the sweating caused by the weight of the fleece would be detrimental to their progress in spite of any amount of extra feeding. It is whispered that exhibitors have been known to "walk round" the rules, by shearing before the prescribed time, repeating the operation, or, at all events, clipping the fleece, at the proper period, to keep within the letter of the law. As soon as the sheep have adapted themselves to the new condition of things, the best possible food is placed before them at intervals of a few hours, and when they have eaten what they choose, the remainder is removed, and they are left undisturbed till the next feeding time. If regularity be observed they soon learn when to look for their meals and rest better during the interval.

For the sake of their general health and appearance, good dry bedding, frequently changed, must be provided, and their feet pared and attended to. With the Down breeds occasional trimming of the fleece is necessary.

Cloths should always be used after shearing, to protect them from cold, and with the short-woolled breeds this is even done after the final trimming and coloring.

WASHINGS—

the first about a month; the second, ten days previous to exhibition—are usually sufficient; tepid water and soap being employed for the purpose. At the finish, the soap must be thoroughly rinsed out of the fleece with clean water. This is only done in the case of certain long wool breeds.

Care must be taken that the wool has had sufficient time to become properly set ere the shears are called into operation for

TRIMMING.

A week, at least, should elapse between washing and trimming—if this precaution is neglected one runs a risk of leaving marks in the fleece which it will be impossible to obliterate afterwards.

In using the shears it is best to bring the animals by slow degrees and repeated trimmings into perfect form. The final trimming is generally given the day previous to exhibition.

In the case of Blackfaced sheep nothing can be done with the shears to improve the appearance of the fleece—washing and *combing* being all that is customary.

Shortwoolled breeds are treated in the same manner as the longwools, save when it is intended to

COLOUR

the fleece, in which case washing is unnecessary unless the wool is very dirty. The fleece is kept close and compact by frequent use of the shears. The colouring material is usually applied a day or two previous to showing.

Various substances are employed for colouring the fleece; the most common being red and yellow ochre, and burnt umber, dissolved in water, or mixed with oil, the shade of colour varying according to the fancy of the owner, and the mixture being rubbed in with a brush. In some instances the following method is adopted :—Ochre and water are mixed to the consistency of stiff paste ; the hands being wetted with olive oil, a little of the paste is rubbed briskly in them until thoroughly mixed with the oil ; the fleece is then carefully gone over with this mixture, which is clapped well into it. In other cases the colouring material is wrought into the wool by means of flat boards (something similar to those used by plasterers), attached to the operator's hands by means of leathern straps.

FATTENING SHOW SHEEP FOR KILLING.

Shows and sales of fat stock are now held at most of the live stock centres throughout the country during the Christmas season, or at other periods of the year.

In most cases sheep intended for these competitions are forced for months with dainties of all sorts, at a total disregard of expense; the endeavour usually being to secure the coveted trophy no matter what outlay is incurred in the attempt. Much the same procedure is adopted as in the case of the summer shows.

One need have little hesitation in saying that were the successful competitors bound to give a detailed and strictly accurate statement of their expenditure, the cost would, in very many cases be found to exceed the profit of the transaction.

The avowed object of all shows is to encourage profitable feeding, but apart from this there can be little doubt that by constantly placing before the farmer the highest class of sheep, and promoting a healthy rivalry among competitors, their general effect is to stimulate the production of finer flocks.

HILL FLOCKS.

MANAGEMENT ON HILL FARMS.

The management of hill farms varies to a considerable extent in different districts, much depending on the nature of the pasture.

In the majority of cases hill farms are so situated that one portion of the land is best fitted for ewes; another part better adapted for hoggs, and the remainder for wedders—the low-lying and best sheltered portion being retained for

the breeding sheep and the more exposed and elevated parts
being allotted to the wedders.

Hill ewes usually have their first lambs when two years
old ; but in some poor, high, and exposed situations, where
they are longer in attaining their full size, they are not
permitted to breed until three years old. Such cases are
however very exceptional, and only three crops are taken
from these ewes. Three or four crops of lambs are generally
taken on the hill before the ewes are cast, or drafted, for
crossing and feeding off.

This crossing is done for the purpose of getting early
lambs which may be quickly got ready for the butcher and
thus enable the ewe to be fattened before the market becomes glutted with ewe mutton.

THE TUPPING SEASON.

The period at which the rams are admitted to the ewes is
regulated by the situation of the farm and nature of the
grazing, care being necessary to arrange matters so that the
lambs may not be dropped until there is likely to be a fair
bite of grass available for the ewes. This is of necessity
dependent upon climatic and local conditions. In the South
of England, and on warm, dry, and early lands, the ram is
put to the ewes as early as August or September, but in the
Northern hilly districts, November is the month usually
chosen, the 22nd being the date selected in many quarters.

On farms abounding with moss, harestail, cotton, and other
early grasses, they may with safety be let free earlier than
in places where these plants are scarce, as they begin growing
with the first appearance of mild weather, and furnish
abundance of food for the sheep until grass becomes plentiful, which, in late and exposed situations, can scarcely be
expected before the end of April. Fifty to sixty ewes are
usually allotted to one ram.

TREATMENT OF RAMS.

Tho rams generally remain with the ewes about two months, and are afterwards kept in an enclosure by themselves, being fed on hay and turnips. In the event of roots being unavailable, a little artificial feeding, such as oilcake and oats may be given to restore their condition. This treatment, among other advantages, is found to ward off inflammatory attacks.

WINTER FEEDING.

Throughout tho winter season hill sheep, in the majority of cases, subsist almost wholly on the poor and scanty diet which their pasturage affords, hay being usually supplied only when the ground is covered with such a depth of snow that it is impossible for the animals to obtain access to the heather and other coarse herbage existing at this season of the year. The sheep work wonderfully to obtain a livelihood when the snow is soft ; but should a partial thaw be succeeded by hard frost, a crust forms on the surface of the snow, and effectually locks the eatables out of their reach.

When it is possible to carry the animals through tho winter in fair condition without having recourse to hand-feeding, it is no doubt advisable to do so for various reasons, not the least important being the saving of expense. The sheep-owner should however be careful that too much scope is not given to his saving propensities. " He that scattereth, gathereth," and it should be ever borne in mind that if it will not pay to keep sheep in reasonably good condition it certainly wont mend matters to half starve them. This is an axiom which applies to sheep-farming everywhere. A good supply of hay should therefore be always at command, sufficient to carry the sheep through the most severe and lasting season.

In feeding with hay, a very common practice is to scatter
it in handfuls on the snow. This method is a very wasteful
one. By erecting a double row of wire or hemp netting, and
stuffing the space betwixt the nets with the hay, the sheep
would have no difficulty in helping themselves through the
meshes, and loss of food would in great measure be prevented.
One to one-and-a-half lb. per head daily is considered a fair
allowance during storms. If no netting is at hand two
hurdles placed so as to form a kind of rack may be used.

SHELTER FOR HILL SHEEP.

In all exposed situations (and the greater number of hill-
farms must be classed under this category), it is important
that shelter should always be available for the flocks during
stormy weather. There is a deal of truth in the old assertion,
"shelter is half meat."

Exposure to the biting blasts of winter has a very hurtful
effect on the animals, leading to a greatly increased death-
rate, and weakening to a considerable extent the constitution
of the survivors.

No better protection can be given than that supplied by
carefully situated plantations, which are however in too
many cases conspicuous only by their absence. Whilst
the provision of this form of shelter would be a boon of
incalculable value to both sheep and sheep-owners, the providing of it is a matter for the owners of the land to deal
with. That it would be to their interest to give more attention than is, in many cases, bestowed upon it is evident,
when we consider that the necessary outlay involved by
planting would in course of time be repaid in two ways—
(1) by the value of the timber itself, and (2) by the increased letting value of the farms. Many, to their own loss,
are quite neglectful of the sage advice, "Aye be stickin' in a
tree, it'll grow when ye are sleeping."

The want of natural woods, or plantations, for sheltering the sheep during violent snow-storms has been in many cases met, by the erection of rough enclosures of circular form, consisting of a wall of dry stone or turf, about five feet high, on portions of the hill known to be least liable to drift.

About the beginning of the present century covered cots were erected in various quarters for sheltering purposes; but, rather unexpectedly, the cure was found to be as bad, if not worse, than the disease. No difficulty was experienced in getting the sheep to take advantage of the shelter thus provided for them; the main trouble lay in getting them, when once in, to venture out in search of food during stormy weather, and, as might be expected, confinement in such warm quarters was found to have a tendency to weaken the constitution of the animals, and so render them less able to withstand subsequent and unavoidable exposure on the hill.

BRATTING.

Sheep can be protected to a very considerable extent from the severity of the weather during winter by "bratting,"—a "brat" being a piece of coarse cloth, or flannel, (rendered waterproof by dipping in boiling tar) sufficiently large to cover the animal's back and ribs, and secured by means of straps, or cords, passed across the breast, behind the shoulders, under the middle of belly, and in front and rear of the hind legs.

Bratting, once pretty general in the case of young sheep, is not much practised nowadays; but there can be no doubt that the custom had much to recommend it. In the case of poor-conditioned sheep bratting would prove specially serviceable, and frequently lower the rate of mortality.

In the Western States of America, where the cold is of extreme severity, it is the practice to "corral" sheep at night during a "cold snap." These corrals, large enough to contain about 2000 sheep, are located on the most protected sites, and usually consist simply of circular fences. The fence "cuts" the biting blast, and the sheep lying closely together, afford mutual warmth, and turn out in the morning none tho worse. The neglect of this simple precaution often involves the loss of no inconsiderable proportion of the flock.

Further notes on this subject will be found on p. 65.

THE LAMBING SEASON.

On hill farms it is customary to allow the ewes the full range of their pasture ground during the lambing season, the same as at other periods of the year. It is, however, desirable that there should be some

ENCLOSURES FOR AILING SHEEP

on the most favourable parts of the ground. In every flock there are sure to be some animals which require special attention—such as ewes having twins, or gimmers that may be careless in looking after their lambs. In such enclosures a shed should be erected, containing a few small pens for the accommodation of ewes that may lose their lambs (and in which it is intended to place others, taken from the ewes that have twins), and ailing animals requiring confinement.

On every hill farm a few

EWE CRIBS

should be reserved in store. These are light wooden enclosures about 5 feet in length, 3 feet in breadth, and 3 feet in height; half-roofed over, and fitted with a small hay-rack and trough for feeding.

In the event of a ewe dropping a weakly lamb on a distant part of the hill, one of these cribs could easily be carried to the spot, and ewe and lamb confined in it as long as might be needful, in place of the shepherd being under the necessity of removing them to the homestead, or leaving them, as is sometimes done, to take their chance, which generally ends in the death of the lamb owing to the ewe deserting it. Failing this the thatched hurdle (p. 66) may be put up with advantage.

TREATMENT OF WEAKLY LAMBS.

The success of hill-lambings, which usually commence about the second or third week of April, depends very much on the state of the weather and condition of the ewes at that period.

When the sheep are in fair condition, and the weather genial, the ewes will have plenty of milk, which renders the shepherd's work comparatively easy, since hill ewes rarely require assistance in lambing, and the lambs are so hardy that with ordinarily mild weather they require little attention. This is fortunate both for shepherd and flock, since owing to the ewes being scattered over the hill it is impossible for the shepherd—no matter how careful and anxious he may be—to give the same attention to them as can be done on lowland farms, where the flocks are smaller in numbers and less scattered.

When the season is backward, grass scarce, and the sheep in poor condition, the shepherd's task is by no means an enviable one. When the weather is cold and wet he will frequently be almost at his wits end as to how best to deal with the number of weakly youngsters that will fall on his hands.

Hill lambs can withstand a wonderful amount of exposure to all appearance unharmed, if only favoured with dry weather for the first few days of their existence, and provided the ewes have a moderate supply of milk. When the latter commodity is scarce, and cold, wet weather prevails, a heavy death-rate is almost certain to be experienced. A favourite means of dealing with lambs suffering from the effects of exposure is to shelter them at a fireside for a short time. A quicker method of restoring them is by immersion in warm water for a few minutes. Lambs brought round thus are usually found weakly in constitution afterwards, and it is far better to place them along with the ewes in some well-sheltered corner, and administer at intervals a little warm milk containing a few drops of whisky or brandy.

DISPOSAL OF HILL STOCK.

After weaning time the stock is disposed of according to the nature of the farm. The best of the ewe-lambs are retained for breeding purposes, and the drafts of them and the wedder lambs are usually sold at this period. The ewe-lambs however are seldom too closely drawn, it being found most profitable to retain a few of the best of the "seconds" to fill up the voids always caused by death. At this period all the lambs intended to be kept on, receive the flock and age marks on the ear, in addition to being buisted with a tar-mark on the side. The "cast" ewes are generally disposed of in the month of October, being bought up by low-ground farmers for breeding cross lambs. In some cases, however, where circumstances are suitable, they are kept on, put to ram, and sold off just previous to lambing.

WINTERING THE HOGGS.

The lambs (or hoggs, as they are then termed,) are generally removed to the lowlands for their first winter, where they have better pasture, and suffer less from exposure than they would do on the hill. They leave home about the beginning of November, and return about the first of April.

In some cases the wedder lambs are wintered on turnips, having an outrun of pasture. Notwithstanding the fact that the sheep on hill farms are not kept in anything like the condition that they are in the lowlands, the expense of these methods of wintering forms a heavy item in the hill-farmer's annual balance sheet.

In some instances the ewe-lambs are wintered along with the ewes; being turned back amongst them two or three weeks after weaning. Where circumstances are favourable for the adoption of this method the system has much to commend it—the lambs being found to be much less liable to fall victims to disease, and the ewes training them to seek both food and shelter. On farms where this practice is followed the ravages of the much-dreaded and fatal disorder known as "braxy," or sickness, are said to have become greatly lessened.

Wedder lambs are weaklier in constitution and more difficult to rear than the ewes; on returning from their winter quarters they are turned to the higher parts of the hill, being disposed of when two or three years old.

VALUATION OF HILL-STOCK.

The ordinary method is to appoint two arbiters, (one being chosen by the outgoing, the other by the incoming tenant), and an oversman, by whom any dispute arising between the arbiters is settled, and whose judgment is final. On a fixed day the stock is gathered together and submitted to the inspection of these judges, who generally decide the value there and then; on some occasions, however, they take the matter to "avizandum," and do not issue their decision until some time afterwards.

After the inspection the stock is counted over to the new tenant.

Sheep bred on the farm are always regarded as being of more value to the incoming tenant than stock purchased at a distance would be, and the value put upon the animals by the valuers is in every instance higher—sometimes very much so—than the prices current in the open market. In

some quarters of the country the fact of the sheep being
acclimatised is of more value than in others. Take Perthshire
for instance—on the great majority of hill farms in that county
the matter would be of little importance. In Argyleshire,
on the contrary, it would be absolutely vital, and any
attempt to stock farms in many parts of that county with
sheep other than those reared on the place, would, in most
cases, prove little less than ruinous to the experimenter.

HILL SHEPHERDING.

The duties of a hill shepherd are by no means so easy as
the uninitiated might suppose.

During the winter months especially, the flocks require
very careful looking after, and even where the greatest
caution is exercised heavy losses will at times occur—sheep
being drowned, overwhelmed in snow drifts, and occasionally
disappearing bodily, in ways impossible to account for.

Shepherds, as a class, are generally regarded as having a
considerable faculty for taking things easily—their work
does not, except at certain seasons, call for the exercise
of much seeming activity, and possibly it is owing to this
that they have had attributed to them the possession of
such an undesirable virtue. If this does exist, it is wholly
due to choice, since there is at all seasons of the year, something or other to which the shepherd can put his hand
which will prove directly or indirectly for the benefit of his
flock.

Fencing is now in many quarters becoming more common,
and lessening the shepherd's duties to a considerable extent
so far as herding the sheep on his own ground is concerned.
Ample scope however exists on most farms for the exercise
of all the shepherd's ingenuity in guiding the members of
his flock so that they may at all seasons of the year be distributed in such a manner that each shall have his, or her,

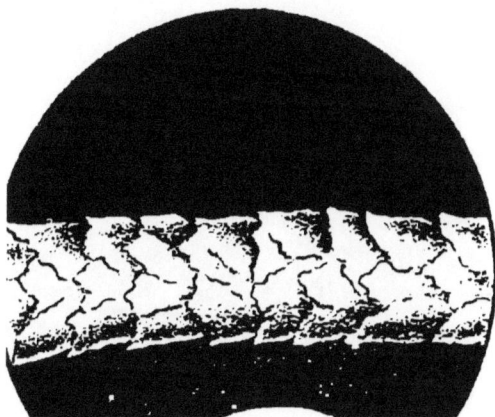

TRANSVERSE SECTION OF WOOL FIBRE.
(Lincoln Hog.) 450 diameters.

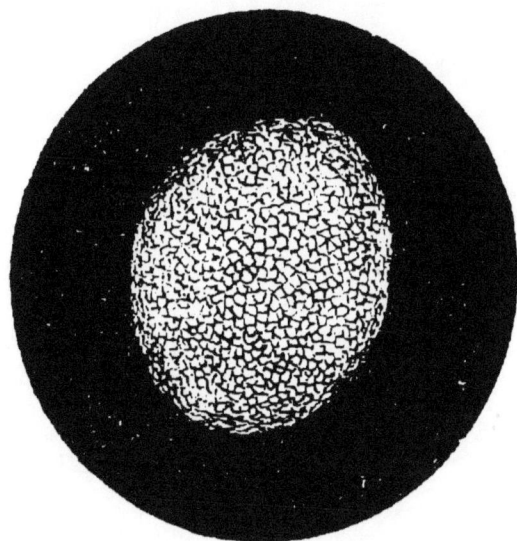

TYPICAL WOOL FIBRE.
250 diameters.

proper share of all the good things going. When left too
much to the freedom of their own will, sheep are very apt to
search out the sweetest spots and neglect the other portions ;
thus injuring the pasture, and probably inducing disease
among themselves.

A great difference exists between the herbage on the
heights and that growing in the hollows, and certain portions
of the pasture may be more valuable for grazing purposes
at one season of the year than at others. A shepherd who
carefully studies all such matters, and carries his knowledge
into practice, is invaluable on a hill farm ; and when such a
treasure is found it is for the employer's own interest to see
that his faithful service does not pass unrequited.

There is one point in which many shepherds err, viz :—in
the too frequent and rash employment of their four-footed
assistants. A deal of harm is done, no doubt thoughtlessly,
in this manner. "Dogging," hurtful to any class of sheep,
is specially so in the case of in-lamb ewes, and serious outbreaks of abortion have been traced to this source.

WOOL.

Unfortunately for the British flockmaster, the value of
wool has fallen very considerably of late years, the immense
quantity received from abroad seriously affecting prices.

Fifty years ago the average quantity annually imported
into Britain was about 26,800 tons. Since then the increase
has been enormous, the average annual imports for the last
five years being 241,300 tons. The quantity re-exported
during the same period averaged 129,720 tons—shewing a
yearly excess of imports over exports of no less than 111,580
tons.

The imported wool, about two-thirds of which hails from
the Australian Colonies, is, as a rule, much superior in
quality to that produced in Britain.

In order to get a better appreciation of the various points of this interesting subject it will be well for the reader to make himself acquainted with the nature, composition, and structure of the fibre.

Structure.—Wool is made up of an infinite number of cells, each fibre having a bulbous root from which the new cells are constantly being developed, each set of cells pushing outward the preceding ones and so producing what we call the growth of the wool.

The accompanying sketches of the fibre magnified illustrate (1), the internal structure showing the cells, and (2), the external form. From the latter it will be seen that the wool is not a smooth hollow sheath, but that its outer covering consists of a series of scales. When the wool is growing, these all point outwards, and therefore cause no inconvenience ; but if the fibre be mingled irrespective of direction, the scales interlock, and this (combined with the wavy character of the wool fibres, which causes them to wrap round each other) occasions matting in parts of the fleece. But these characteristics have a very great value from a commercial point of view, for it is by their aid that the felting process in cloth making is accomplished.

The Yolk.—When the wool is growing, a quantity of unctuous fatty matter is secreted from the skin. This is called the yolk, and there is no doubt it exercises an important function in softening the wool and preserving the surface "scales" from injury. It is a certain fact that the best wool is grown where the yolk is most abundant. The Merino fleece is a case in point. So largely does this yolk enter into the economy of wool growing that in the Merino it constitutes 33 per cent. of the weight of the fleece, the actual fibre being only 31 per cent. or less than one third of its weight when shorn.

Chemical composition.—This varies slightly in the different breeds of sheep, as the following table from analysis by Dr. Bowman* will show.

	Lincoln Wool.	Irish Wool.	Northumberland Wool.	Southdown Wool.
Carbon	52.0	49.8	50.8	51.3
Hydrogen	6.9	7.2	7.2	6.9
Nitrogen	18.1	19.1	18.5	17.8
Oxygen	20.3	19.9	21.2	20.2
Sulphur	2.5	3.0	2.3	3.8
Loss	0.2	1.0	—	—
	100.0	100.0	100.0	100.0

It is a singular fact that these analysis are almost identical with those of hair, feathers, nails, claws, horns, hoofs, and scales of other animals, and this gives strong support to the contention now generally accepted by scientists that these appendages are nothing more than modified developments of hair.

Density of the fleece.—Fineness of fibre almost invariably governs the degree in which the wool curves, and also the density of the fleece. There are fifteen times more curves in the Merino than in the Lincoln wool. Hence the relatively increased value of the former for felting purposes.

The Leicester will carry from 1500 to 1900 fibres per square inch on the shoulder, the South Down 2000 to 2500, while the Merino will be much greater.

Matters affecting growth of Wool.—Such a complex and delicate structure as the wool, is naturally influenced by the surroundings or environment of the sheep. A comparison of flocks of similar breed will shew that the heaviest and finest qualities of wool are produced on good land, and where

* "Structure of the Wool Fibre," p. 170. Published by Palmer & Howe, Princes Street, Manchester.

the sheep are well cared for, kept clean in the skin, and in a constantly thriving state. On poor and exposed farms, and where the animals are neglected, and infested with insects, or kept in a half-starved state, the yolk is deficient in quantity, and the wool is of an inferior quality, being harsh, short, and brittle ; and occasionally becomes so matted, (particularly if long-continued wet weather prevail,) as to be almost useless for manufacturing purposes.

The nature of the soil determines the properties of the pasture, and thereby influences the quality of the wool—but this influence is, of course modified by the quality and breed of the sheep.

There can be no doubt that a persistent diet of food containing larger proportions of the wool-producing substances would have a material effect upon the fleece.

It is rather unfortunate, however, that as a rule the best wool breeds are the worst meat producers. The Merino has a small carcase, but its fleece frequently exceeds 30 lbs. in weight. The fleece of the Lincoln is perhaps one fourth, and the carcase in almost inverse ratio.

Every flockmaster having regard to the welfare of his flocks, should bear in mind that the wool is a daily and hourly barometer of the life of the sheep. If they suffer, so does the wool, and although a temporary check to the "condition" of the flock may be made up, the weakness in the fibre which it has brought about can never be removed. The healthier the animal, the better and more regular the wool at shearing. Sheep infected with ticks or other parasites grow neither as much meat or wool as clean animals. A sudden change in feeding, or condition, immediately tells its tale in the cells which are always building up the new wool. This produces a weakness and sometimes a distinct break in

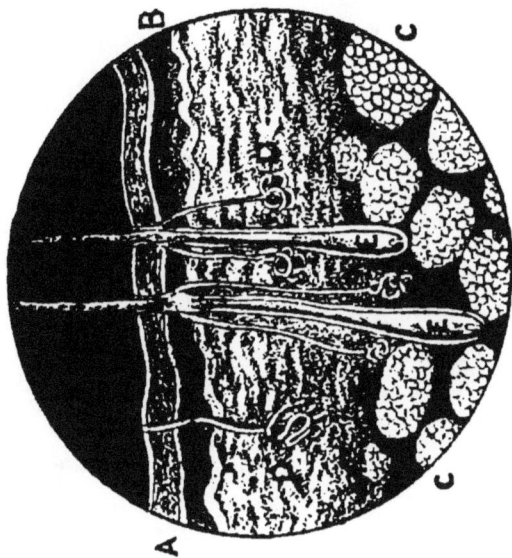

SECTION OF SKIN. 25 diameters.

A The two outer layers (the epidermis).
B "   "   inner   "   (the dermis).
C Fat cells.
D Sweat and yolk glands.
E Roots of wool.

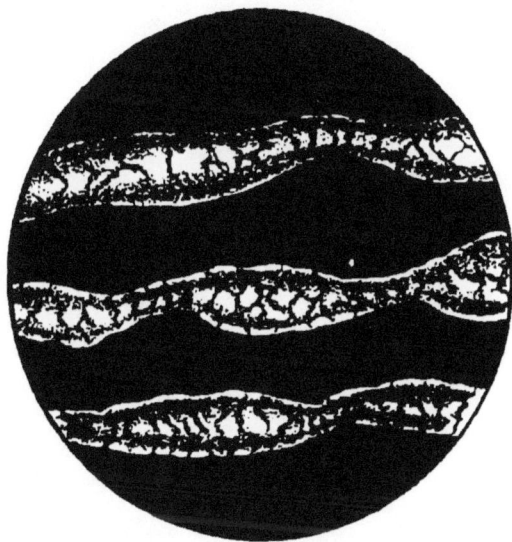

DISEASED WOOL.
Magnified.

the fibre, quite usual with an attack of scab. Dipping with such of the so-called non-poisonous compounds as check the condition of the sheep has the same tendency.

Among the Savage Races the "knowledge that starvation produced a deterioration of the fibre was turned to account, before the introduction of shearing, as a means of obtaining the fleece from the sheep. The animals were confined without food for some days until a short growth of weak and debilitated hair had been produced, and thus the fleece could readily be torn from the surface of the skin."

It is a mistake to suppose that all the wool would be shed if no shearing took place. In countries where it is difficult to ensure the complete mustering of the sheep, they are sometimes found with wool of enormous length, though there is always a "break" or weakness to show each year's growth. The finest and most evenly grown portions of the wool are always on the shoulders, and the coarsest on the hind legs.

The finest British wool is produced by the Down, the coarsest by the Long Wools and Hill Breeds.

[We are indebted to Dr. Bowman, Author of "The Structure of the Wool Fibre," for many of the facts contained in this article, and also for the illustrations of wool.]

SHEEP SORTING PENS AND YARDS.

Nearly every field on which sheep are grazing should be provided with a pen into which they can be run when any of them require handling. There is nothing worse than hunting and dogging them into corners when it is necessary to get hold of any of them.

For temporary pens, flakes or hurdles answer fairly well and have the advantage, when one patch of ground has become foul, of being readily removable to a fresh clean place ; but on every farm where a regular stock of sheep is kept, a

substantial and conveniently arranged drawing pen should be
erected near the homestead.

The colonial "race," or method of drawing sheep is a very
efficient one. They are driven into a large pen, the exit
passage from which is usually 3 or 4 yards in length, 18 or
20 inches in width, and the sides (which are close lined,)
3½ feet in height. At the far end of this passage two other
pens are situated, the fence dividing them running in a
parallel line with the centre of the passage. A light gate is
attached to the fence at the end of the passage, so as to be
easily swung to either side by the party in charge of it, that
the sheep may be run into either of the pens as desired.
When the sheep are once got in motion up the passage
they can be separated into two lots with great rapidity. By
lengthening the exit passage and hanging extra gates so as to
give access to other side pens, the flock can be separated into
as many lots as may be needful.

The exit passage is very useful when drawing out fat
sheep for sale, as, when filled up, by closing each end of it,
the shepherd can handle each animal carefully with ease to
himself and without harassing the sheep in the least. Those
for disposal can be "keel marked" in the passage, and
afterwards run into a pen by themselves.

CASTRATING AND DOCKING.

Advantage should always, if possible, be taken of a moist,
showery day, which is much more favourable for the operation than dry weather. A close and sultry day should be
avoided.

The operation should be performed when the lambs are
comparatively young, as at that stage they evidently suffer
less pain, and less risk of loss is incurred than when the
operation is deferred until the animals are more forward in

size and condition. Two or three weeks after birth is about the usual period chosen—a few days more or less makes little difference.

The whole operation should be conducted as quietly and gently as possible, since if the animals are put into an excited or heated state, there is always a risk, or indeed it may be said almost a certainty, of loss being experienced. The ewes and lambs should be gathered into the fold and the former drawn out; when they have settled down operations may be commenced.

The shepherd will require two assistants—one to catch the lambs and the other to hold them in proper position. He should also have two knives at hand—the finest and sharpest blade being retained for castrating.

The party holding the lamb should keep the animal with its back firmly pressed against his left shoulder, grasping a fore and hind foot in each hand, (but not so tightly together as to make the belly concave). Drawing the testicles back, the shepherd cuts off the tip of the scrotum, or bag; presses with both hands on the abdomen so as to start the testicles, which he then draws out singly with his teeth. Occasionally the thumb and fore-finger of the left hand are employed in place of the teeth, but the latter make the most rapid and satisfactory work.

In some instances a different course is adopted—the testicles being pressed forward by the left hand to the tip of the scrotum, two cuts are made through the integuments opposite the testicles (in place of cutting off the very tip), and they are then drawn out. ,

This latter system is, however, open to serious objection, since in many cases the wounds heal up so rapidly that should suppuration set in no outlet is left for pus, and dangerous inflammation ensues. By adopting the former method all discharges are easily got rid of, as the wound takes longer to heal up.

A very rough method of castration is practised in some parts of America—the scrotum and testicles being severed at one stroke close to the belly by means of a pair of strong sheep-shears. The operation is performed when the lambs are only a few days old, and is said to ensure the best results. Another way, and one often employed when lambs are older, is for an assistant to hold the lamb while the operator, after removing the tip of the scrotum, presses out the testicles with his thumb and finger, and removes them with a hot iron made for the purpose; afterwards searing the end of the cord to prevent hæmorrhage.

Immediately after castration, a little of a mixture of carbolic acid and olive oil—1 part to 20—should be applied to the wound. This is one of the very best applications for the purpose, preventing inflammation and arresting excessive bleeding. Before letting the lamb free the tail should be sharply pulled once or twice, so as to replace the disarranged chords and vessels.

After castration the lambs should be carefully "mothered," as, owing to the pain they experience, they are apt to lie down and pay no attention to the bleating of the ewes, and if once fairly separated they may not readily find each other again.

The losses sometimes experienced after castration may, I think, in most cases be attributed to one of three causes :—

(1.) To hæmorrhage or bleeding after the operation.

(2.) To the animals having been unduly excited just prior to the operation, or being out of health.

(3.) To the results of unsuitable weather.

The tail is generally "docked" or shortened immediately after castration, by one stroke with a sharp knife; in other cases (and this is preferable) the operation is deferred for a week or two longer.

Docking is in some instances carried to extremes, especially by some breeders of the " Down " varieties of sheep. There should be a medium in all things.

WASHING OF SHEEP.

A good deal of uncertainty prevails amongst farmers as to whether it is, or is not, to their advantage to wash their sheep before clipping. Washed wool undoubtedly commands a higher price than unwashed, and the problem (which each grower should be best able to solve for himself)˙therefore is—"Does the extra price received for washed wool recompense one for the loss of weight sustained by, and the expense incurred in, washing?"

There are very many matters that affect the quality of wool, apart altogether from the fact of its being in a washed or unwashed state, and it seems to me that the only satisfactory method of determining whether it does or does not pay to wash is by experimenting on sheep of the same class, and which have all along been treated exactly alike as regards feeding, &c. To argue that washing pays because one lot of *unwashed* wool from one quarter only realised 8½d. per lb., while a *washed* lot from another district brought 1s. 2d. per lb., is perfectly absurd.

It would certainly not be in the wool grower's interests to send the unwashed wool into market just as it came from the animal's body. The fleece should be carefully divested of all stained wool about the breech ; and all dirty and loose tufts about the belly should also be removed, and sold separately. Care should also be taken throughout the year that the sheep do not get the fleece filled with hay-seeds, straw, or other objectionable substances, which would seriously detract from its value.

Where washing is customary, the manner in which the operation is conducted varies according to the size of the flock and the facilities that may be available for the purpose.

On arable farms where the flocks are, as a rule, small in numbers, hand-washing is mostly practised. If a slow-flowing streamlet of sufficient depth exists in the neighbourhood, it is generally taken advantage of for the purpose. An ordinary mill-pond answers very well, provided the bottom be of a gravelly nature.

The sheep being penned on the bank close to the water, two or three men take up positions in the water, a few yards from each other. The sheep are thrown in singly, and passed from one hand to another up stream, leaving the shepherd's hands last—his duty being to see that the washing has been properly carried out before the animals are allowed to swim to the bank. In other instances tank-washing is practised, a small quantity of soap being sometimes added to the bath.

In the case of large flocks either of these methods would prove too tedious for general practice, and swimming is therefore the most common method adopted; the sheep being compelled to pass repeatedly through some convenient pool, on a river, or mountain streamlet. Usually the sheep are enclosed in a large pen, formed of hurdles, the outlet from which consists of a narrow passage. Here the animals are put in motion and compelled to leap into the pool. After their " header," they swim to land as best they can— the operation being repeated as often as may be thought needful.

A careful shepherd, with the assistance of two good dogs, can in this manner thoroughly wash a large number of sheep in a very short time,

The early part of the day is the best period for washing, as the fleece has then time to dry up ere "the shades of evening" fall; and the animals will consequently enjoy a more comfortable night's repose than they would do were their compulsory ablutions deferred till later in the day.

After being washed, the sheep should be confined on clean pasture until shorn—this operation being usually performed about a week or ten days after washing.

SHEARING.

As already stated shearing is generally deferred for a week or more after washing; this delay being for the purpose of allowing the fleece to recover in some measure the "yolk," without which the wool would be deficient in brightness and weight, and more difficult to shear.

On hill farms it is (or at least was, not very many years ago—the fashion is dying out now in some quarters) customary for neighbours to assist each other at shearing time—the shepherds on six or eight farms uniting their strength and shearing the flocks on each farm in succession. This system is beneficial in various ways; the clipping of even the largest flocks being got over in a few days, in place of taking weeks, as it would do were none engaged at it but the shepherds belonging to the place. The sheep are also less harassed—less gathering and dogging being required.

These annual meetings are also serviceable in enabling the shepherds to regain possession of any wandering members of their flocks, which may have strayed from their respective farms.

The time for this operation also varies according to climate and other conditions. In the South of England it commences about the beginning of May, becoming later as we travel northwards. The hoggs are generally shorn first, the ewes two or three weeks afterwards.

In the open country, to save re-gathering the flock, each sheep as soon as it is shorn is stamped, or "buisted" with the flock-mark—usually the initials of the owner's name. A considerable amount of trouble is sometimes experienced in getting the lambs properly mothered after the ewes are clipped, the latter being so altered in appearance on having the fleece removed that the youngsters fail to recognise them. The shepherd requires to give careful attention to this matter, otherwise weaning may take place rather too early in the season.

METHODS OF SHEARING.

The methods of shearing are equally varied. On hill farms in Scotland the work is usually conducted in the open air ; the sheep being placed before the shepherds on turf seats. The wool on the belly is first removed ; the animals legs are then tied together with soft cord, and the shears run rapidly over the body, longways, from head to tail. Hill sheep, as a rule, are very roughly clipped ; this however is not considered objectionable, since the roughness left on the skin tends to protect the animals during inclement weather, which is frequently experienced on high and exposed farms, even at this advanced period of the year.

The sheep are confined in pens close beside the clipping ground, one man catching for eight or ten clippers.

The fleece, on being removed from the sheep, is (or, at all events, should be,) freed from all extraneous matter,—all stained wool being removed—and then rolled neatly and firmly up, and tied with a band twisted from the neck end of the fleece.

On Scottish hill farms—more particularly those in the northern counties—the cleaning and tying up of the wool is usually entrusted to females.

On lowland farms, shearing, when not performed by the

shepherd himself, is generally carried out by piece-work—
the rate of pay varying according to the size and class of
sheep; an ordinary allowance, for the white-faced classes,
being 2d. to 3d. per head. Lowland sheep are seldom clipped
longways, being generally shorn round the ribs; and the
animals not being so easily handled as the lighter hill sheep,
are usually clipped on the ground (a clean pasture field being
chosen for the operation), their legs being left untied. In
some instances shearing is carried on under cover—the
straw-barn, or other suitable outhouse, being selected for the
purpose.

CARE OF THE FLEECE.

The fleece should be removed as whole as possible; when
it gets tumbled about and broken it reduces the value.

In most cases the fleece is rolled up on the grass. This
system is, however, open to objection; as it is scarcely
possible in such cases to keep the wool free from dirt. By
spreading it on a sparred platform raised a short distance
from the ground, all earth and other adhering matter falls
clear of the fleece in the process of folding and rolling.

Blackfaced wool is usually tied with the weather side of
the fleece out: all other classes with the white side exposed.

The wool should be carefully packed and sewn up, in
sacks or sheets, immediately after shearing; and, if not then
sent off to market, placed in a dark, cool, dry, and vermin-
proof storehouse. A hot and well-lighted storeroom is very
objectionable, as the wool becomes scorched, loses lustre,
and diminishes considerably in weight.

In packing the wool in sheets—which are generally sus-
pended by ropes from the couples of the wool-room in such
a position that the bottom of the pack almost touches the
flooring—the fleeces should be placed in layers, alternately
cross-ways and lengthways, and firmly trampled down.

DRAFTING.

The flockmaster should be a proficient in the art of weeding. He who annually overhauls his flock, and drafts from it with no niggard hand all the faulty and likely-to-be-unprofitable members, is certain, at the year's end, to show a much more favourable balance-sheet than the one who neglects this point. The farmer's motto should be "the best of everything," and, no matter what class of stock is kept—be it breeding, feeding, or store—the endeavour should always be to retain only really good sheep ; as they always turn out the most profitable in the end.

In the case of a breeding flock, thorough weeding is specially desirable. All old broken-mouthed ewes, those that are faulty in udder, deficient in milking properties, or other important respects, or that have proved uncertain breeders—all such may be classed as "unprofitable servants," and should be got rid of at the earliest favourable opportunity.

SMEARING.

The practice of *smearing*, or "salving" as it was at first termed, has been traced back to the time of the ancient Romans ; but whether the custom originated with them is now unknown. The mixture they employed was a rather formidable one—consisting, as it did, of oil, litharge, sulphur, pitch, wax, squills, helebore, and bitumen.

It is not definitely known when the practice was first resorted to in Britian ; but the custom is said to have been introduced from Spain, where the shepherds were in the habit of employing honey, mixed with the essence of various bitter herbs, for the purpose. On its introduction into this country, however, a radical change was made in the composition of the smearing mixture—tar and grease being substituted for the substances used in "the sunny South." The alteration might be mainly due to two causes—honey would no doubt be a scarce commodity in this country, and it might also be thought that tar and grease would be better fitted for withstanding the wetness and changeableness of the British climate. Until the beginning of the present century smearing was customary both amongst high and low ground flocks—save in some cases where pouring was practised.

About the period mentioned dipping began to be resorted to in various quarters, and, although the substances made use of were possibly not of the most suitable kinds, the dipped sheep were found, even in high and exposed situations, to stand the winter's exposure equally as well as those which had been smeared. For a long time afterwards, however, the practice of dipping made little progress. Rooted habits and dislike of new-fangled methods have always proved barriers to the rapid spread of improved systems, and to the strong regard held by farmers for old customs must no doubt be attributed in great measure the long-continued adherence in many quarters to the practice of smearing. Within the last twenty years, however, this old method has been rapidly giving way in favour of the new, and dipping may now be said to be almost universally practised.

Compared with the modern method, smearing was a slow and costly process, and in addition it also lessened the value of the wool considerably.

Smearing was considered by many as tending to promote warmth during the winter season, and it may have had a tendency to do so in the case of conditioned sheep; but one would be apt to think that the practice would have an entirely contrary effect in the case of lean animals—the weight of the smearing composition being likely to cause the fleece to open along the back; and so expose the frame of the animals to, instead of protecting it from, the cold and wet.

Once the rain makes its way down between the skin and the waterproofing material on the fleece, which it always does, the animals must be in anything but a comfortable state until the moisture gets dried up by the heat of their bodies.

Passing, however, from by-gones, we may now deal directly with our subject :—

DIPPING.

Objects of Dipping.—The majority of sheepmen dip for the destruction of parasites, such as the Scab Insect, Ticks, Lice, and Maggots. This, however, is only one of many advantages to be derived from the operation.

The benefit of a perfect dip will remain in the fleece for months, killing the young insects as they are hatched, warding off subsequent attacks, and contributing to · the growth and quality of the wool. When these objects are achieved the outlay is returned tenfold.

A few years ago it was the exception rather than the rule to dip. Now any farmer who neglects to do so at least once a year is a curiosity rarely met with.

When to Dip.—The best time for the ordinary dipping is from one or two months after shearing, for at that time the wool is sufficiently long to hold all the wash required and not long enough to carry off an unnecessary quantity. At this time also it is the greatest protection against Maggot-fly. In many districts an Autumn dipping is also carried out. Experience has shown this to be a very paying investment, and the time is not far distant when the second dipping will become general. Nobody who has watched the difference between a dipped flock grazing undisturbed, and resting in comfort, and an undipped one, never at rest, can doubt it. The prices of the London Wool Market tell the same tale.

Exceptional dippings may profitably take place at any time to meet special circumstances, such as an outbreak of Scab.

Of course care must at all times be taken to avoid unsuitable weather, such as intense heat or cold, which might throw them back in condition. Wet weather is decidedly to be avoided, for when the wool is damp it cannot absorb a sufficient quantity of dip, and if just after dipping, before the fleece has had time to dry, a heavy rain comes on, the solution may in some measure be washed out.

Sheep newly purchased, whatever the time of the year, should be dipped immediately on arrival at the farm. Scab probably breaks out more often through failure to do this than from any other cause.

What Dip to use.—The dip selected should be the one which best accomplishes all the objects possible in dipping. These are as already stated, the destruction of all parasites and their young as they are hatched, the protection from further attack, the like protection from Maggot-fly, and the improvement of the wool. A dip that fails in any one of these objects should be discarded. Regard should also be had to portability, ease in mixing and applying, safety and cheapness, and it should be absolutely uniform in strength.

Many dips actually soil and injure the wool, or throw back the condition of the sheep, or even both. The effects of all carbolic and non-poisonous dips are of a very transient nature. They may—even in this respect many of them fail, unless used at double their directed strength—kill the insects alive in the fleece at the time of dipping; but they are utterly worthless for destroying the eggs present, from which future generations of parasites will spring ; and, unless the sheep are dipped a second time, after an interval of about ten days, the animals will soon be discovered as badly infested with vermin as they were previous to dipping being performed. For summer dipping—to ward off the attacks of the Maggot-fly—carbolic dips seem to me to be *worse than useless.* My experience of them being that they actually attract the flies to the sheep on which they have been used, instead of repelling them.

Other Dips, though prepared by those calling themselves "qualified" men, are mere mechanical mixtures. To this class belong some of the powder dips with which the market is flooded. They fail in most of the essentials of a good dip. Others again are bulky, more or less difficult to mix, require hot water for use, and have an awkward habit of leaking, or varying their character by chemical precipitation—these are of a liquid or pasty nature.

Home-made dips and preparations with pitch-oil require no condemnation from me, as no flockmaster having any regard for the welfare of his sheep would think of using them. Cheapness is the only advantage even claimed for them. I am convinced from a long practical experience that they are dear at any price. They damage the wool, are uncertain as to strength, and have other serious defects.

The making of a perfect dip is a long and complicated process which can only be properly carried out by those having a thorough knowledge of the chemical nature of the ingredients, and the indispensable and costly appliances for their treatment. What then should be the nature and form of these ingredients ? It is perfectly clear that no dip of a non-poisonous character can accomplish all the objects we desire, and to liquid and paste dips of all kinds there are many objections. This is why the judgment of the sheep-

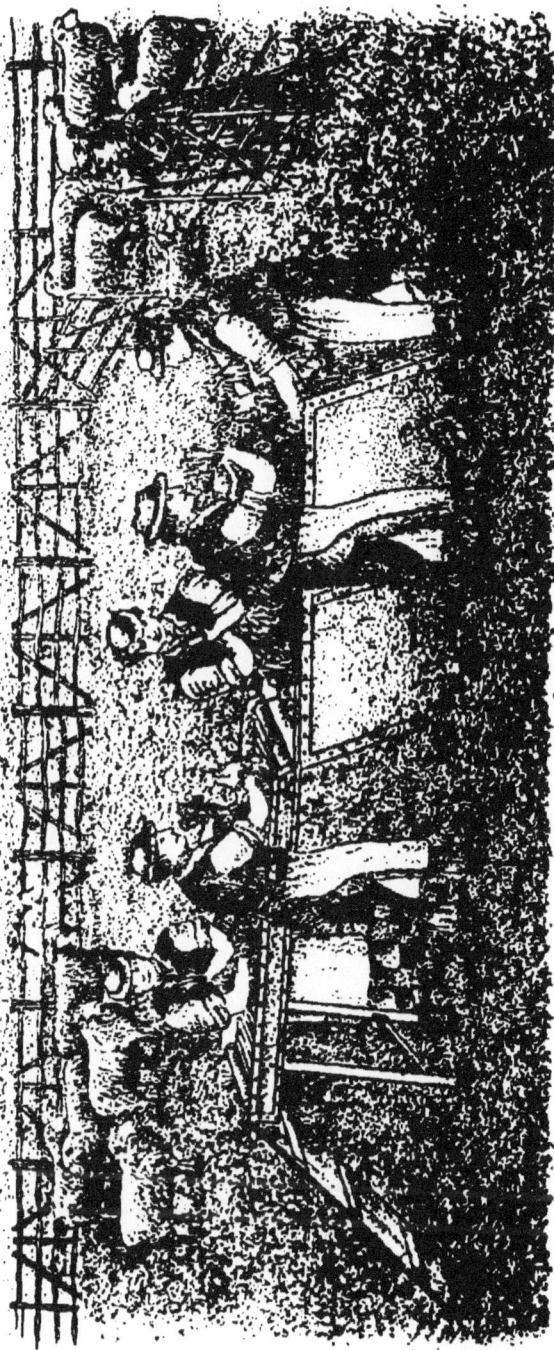

Manufactured by the Proprietors of "Cooper's Dipping Powder."

IRON DIPPING APPARATUS. Drawn by Wm. Cooper & Nephews.

men throughout the world has ranged itself so unmistakably
on the side of the poisonous powder Dip, and has naturally
selected the original of such, viz :—Cooper's Dipping Powder,
of which the others are imitations, in which judgment my
experience has led me to concur.

Mode of Dipping.—The safest advice under this head is to
follow carefully the printed directions issued with the particular dip employed. It is wonderful how careless many
people are with their dipping. They neglect to mix properly,
to stir the bath, or to time the operation, and then expect to
destroy the parasites which lie well protected at the roots of
the wool, and needless to say they are disappointed.

The better plan will perhaps be to quote the instructions
given by a celebrated firm of dip makers—

Mix thoroughly.

Use the right proportion of water.

Keep the bath stirred.

Keep the sheep moving in the bath one minute by the
watch.

With the right dip, failure is then practically impossible.

In cases of scab, a second dipping should take place to
destroy any insects that may have hatched from eggs buried
beneath the skin so as to be beyond the reach of the first dip.
This latter should be done from 14 to 20 days after the first.
If it takes place sooner than this, some eggs may remain
unhatched, and if left later, the newly-hatched insects may
have already begun in their turn to deposit eggs.

Scab being extremely contagious it is advisable not to
return sheep to the infected pasture for at least 3 months,
and as far as practicable all posts, fences, &c., against which
they have been rubbing should be washed with the remedy.

DIPPING APPARATUS.

The baths in use for dipping purposes are almost as

various as the dips themselves. Where the flocks are small
the dipping is usually done in a tub or tank into which the
sheep are lifted as shown in the illustration. As it is impossible for them while in this position to eject any wash
which may get into their mouths, a man is told off to keep
their heads out of the liquid.

They should be briskly moved about to enable the wash
to thoroughly penetrate to the skin, and then lifted on to
the drainer; the bulk of the wash is then pressed out of the
fleece by the hand and finds its way back to the bath.
Heavy rams and ewes in lamb may stand in the bath, and
have the remedy poured over and well rubbed into them,
but this system should be avoided as much as possible, and
only adopted with great care. Even then it is never so
satisfactory as dipping.

The illustration is by the Proprietors of Cooper's Dipping
Powder, who make the apparatus in considerable numbers.

The sheep on leaving the drainer should be turned for at
least an hour or two into an enclosure which is devoid of
pasture or other feeding substances.

Dipping Machines of various designs on wheels are occasionally met with, and are in common use in Lincolnshire
and one or two other localities. A few of these answer fairly
well, whilst others are extremely clumsy and inconvenient,
but against them all is the serious objection that the outlay
is out of all proportion to their efficiency. Seldom costing
less than £25 or £30, the best of them fail to dip more than
700 or 800 sheep in a day, and they are in need of constant
repairs. It is a very old practice in many districts to sink
the hand-dipping bath into the ground, an excavation being
made on either side in which the men stand. The sheep are
taken from a pen at one end, and after being dipped are
raised into a draining pen at the other end.

HOW TO BUILD A SWIMMING BATH.

These suggestions, the result of practical experience in all parts of the world, are only intended to convey some general idea of a suitable bath.
The details can of course be varied to suit individual requirements and materials procurable.

GROUND PLAN.

SECTION.

A Mustering enclosure, into which sheep to be dipped are collected.

B B Pens, by means of which the sheep are conveyed a few at a time from the mustering enclosure to the small internal pen C, from which men pass them quietly into the bath.

K Decoy pen in which a few sheep are placed, to induce the others to enter C.

D D The bath or swim 50 to 60 feet long, 5 feet deep, 9 inches of which must be above the ground level to keep dirt or rubbish out of the bath; 21 inches wide till 3 feet from top, then gradually narrowing to 6 or 8 inches wide at bottom, as shown in section G. For ten feet along the side, at the entrance end of the bath, fix a board or piece of masonry M, 3 feet high to catch the splash. 16 feet from the exit end of the bath the bottom should rise gradually, with ribbed foot-holds, to the level of the draining pens as shown in section H; this will greatly assist the sheep in getting out. To avoid constant measuring of water, it is well to have an upright board fixed in the side of the bath, plainly marked for every 100 gallons, so as to indicate at a glance the point to which the bath must be filled on replenishing.

E E The draining pens. These are filled alternately by means of a swing gate F, which serves for both pens. Each pen should measure not less than 24 feet by 18 feet. The floors must be water-tight, and made sloping towards the bath D, so as to conduct all drippings into it. A narrow perforated ledge, or some such simple contrivance fixed at the top of the sloping end of the bath D will prevent manure being carried back into it with the drippings.

J Cratch for plunging the sheep; it can also be used to assist any that are too weak to swim. It should be 5 to 6 feet long, with a head made of ⅜-inch iron bar. Two or three of these are required.

N Mixer, for stirring the bath. It is made of a stout piece of board about 10 inches long by 8 inches wide with a handle about 6 to 7 feet long, fixed in its centre, and strengthened with side supports as shown. Plunge it down quickly *right on to the bottom* of the bath, and then draw it *nearly up.* This should always be done just before beginning to dip, also after every stoppage and fresh mixing.

The Swim Bath.—By far the most speedy, convenient, effective, and economical method of dipping, however, is by the swimming bath. This is usually a long narrow trench lined with wood, brickwork, or some waterproof material to contain the wash, through which the sheep are made to swim. The accompanying illustration gives full particulars as to its size and construction. The advantages that a long narrow bath, such as this, have over a wider and shorter one are many ; in it the sheep pass through in a regular line, so that each one gets exactly the same time ; and moreover they spend this time in the exertion of swimming, a splendid means of working the remedy through the fleece. The sheep to be dipped should be made to face the bath, their haunches placed on its edge and the body be allowed to fall gently forward, and on their passage through the trench the heads of each one should be once or twice steadily pushed under by means of a crook or forked stick. The exit end of the trench is arranged in the shape of a flight of narrow steps, up which the sheep can walk into a draining pen, where they should be allowed to stand until all surplus wash has escaped from the fleece. The floor of this pen may be made with wood, cement, asphalte, brick, or galvanised iron, and should be so built that all the drippings run back to the trench. It will be found most convenient to divide it into two parts, with a gate so arranged at the exit of the bath that the sheep can come into whichever pen is required. If it be built for each part to contain 200 sheep, and they are filled alternately, every sheep has good time to drain before going on to the pasture.

This bath (the design of which is by Messrs. Cooper and Nephews) is used throughout the Colonies and North and South America—almost everywhere in fact, but in Britain ; and with it as many as 10,000 sheep have been dipped in a

single day. We fear it must be confessed that we are in this
respect very much behind our sheep-farming brethren in the
rest of the world.

The same firm have also introduced a square swimming
bath, which is possibly even better suited to our small flocks
than the long one, inasmuch as less dip is required to fill it,
and there is less waste when the bath is emptied. It can be
made either portable or fixed. In the former case wood or
iron may be used, but if intended as a fixture bricks set in
cement are strongly recommended. Just enough of the bath
should be above the ground to keep dirt and rubbish from
getting kicked in.

Fig. 1 gives a side view, and fig. 2 the view looking into
it. A convenient size is 4-ft. 6-in. deep, 5-ft. square at the
top, narrowing to 4-ft. at the bottom. The exit slope and the
draining pens are the same as in the long swim.

With this bath about 1500 sheep can be easily dipped in
the day. It will hold three sheep at a time, and a man with
a crutch is in charge to see that the animals remain in the
proper time and leave in the right order.

It is probable that this bath will come to be very largely
used in the United Kingdom, as its cost in brick and cement,
exclusive of the draining pen, is less than £5, and it does
its work splendidly. It would certainly be a paying investment for any farmer with a flock of 500 sheep, as it is a
means of enabling this important operation to be done
speedily and cheaply whenever it may appear desirable.

SHEEP MARKING.

In the case of hill-flocks, four systems of marking are
followed—*i.e.*—ear-marking, buisting, keeling, and branding.

Ear-marking.—The ears are generally the recipients of
the age and stock-marks, which in most cases are put on the
lambs at time of weaning.

COOPER'S SQUARE SWIMMING BATH.

Fig. 2.

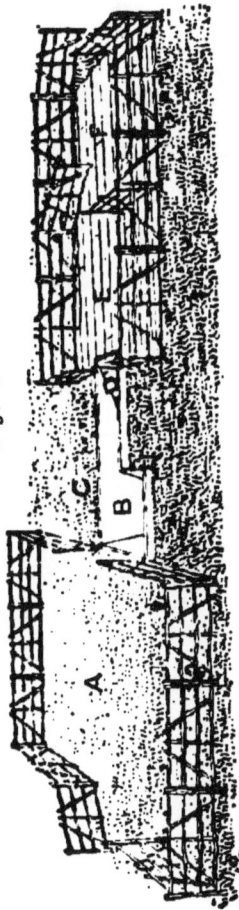

Fig. 1.

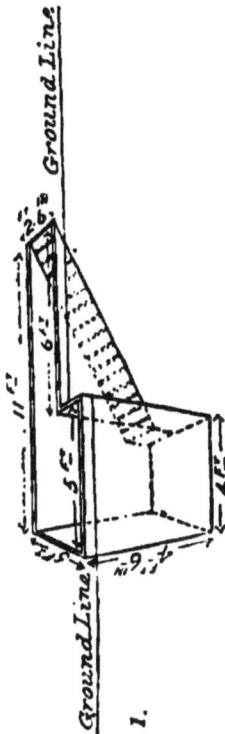

A bath this size will hold three sheep.

A Mustering enclosure into which the sheep to be dipped are collected.

B The bath into which the sheep are passed singly. A man stands at C with a crook to keep the sheep under control, and see that they remain the proper time in the liquid and leave in the order they entered. The exit D should be ribbed so as to give the sheep foothold.

E F The Draining Pens. When E is filled the sheep are passed on to F where they continue draining until E is refilled, when they are turned out. Each pen should be large enough to hold not less than 50 sheep.

The floors should be of brick and cement or corrugated iron, and should be made slightly sloping from the top towards the bath, to conduct the drippings back to the bath.

The *age marks* are usually made by nipping a small piece out of the back or fore margin of the ear, by means of nippers specially manufactured for the purpose—in other cases slits are formed by means of a sharp pocket knife. The number of age-marks employed varies, of course, according to the age at which the sheep are "drafted." If this is done at five years old, five different marks will be required. All this however is quite unnecessary, as the age can be much more reliably obtained from the teeth.—See the article on 'Dentition.'

The *stock mark* generally consists of a small hole, cut in a particular part of one of the ears. All such marks, although they should be made perfectly distinct, ought also to be of small size, otherwise they detract from the appearance of the sheep.

Buist, brand, and keel marks.—In the case of stray sheep, it would be a tedious and difficult job for the shepherd, had he, when searching for stray members of his flock, to examine the ear-marks of all the sheep he might fall in with resembling his own. The use of buist and keel marks obviates this difficulty, in addition to giving a double clue to the ownership, and renders the sheep capable of being distinguished at a considerable distance.

The *buist mark*, which is put on the sheep immediately after they are shorn, usually consists of the initial letter, or letters, of the owner's name,—the stamp being formed of stout sheet-iron, attached to a handle about two feet in length. Boiling tar, or pitch, or a mixture of the two, is the substance generally employed.

The *keel mark*, made by a mixture of red ochre and oil, is put on the sheep about the end of Autumn, as by that period the tar mark becomes very indistinct, owing to the growth of the wool. In some instances, but very seldom, in order the

readier to distinguish the sheep of the various ages, the tar
and keel marks are placed on different parts of the body,
according to the age of the animals. This practice should
be condemned as it leads to confusion. Every sheep-owner
should have his distinct mark, and always have it put upon
the same part of the body.

Branding.—This method of marking is generally adopted
in the case of horned sheep,—the initials of the owner's
name and the year of the animal's birth, being branded on
the horn, by means of red-hot iron dies, or stamps. At one
time it was customary in some quarters to brand the sheep
on the nose, by means of a hot iron, but that barbarous
custom is now rarely practised.

In the case of arable-land flocks, the buist and keel marks
are the most commonly used,—ear-marking being seldom
practised save in the case of breeding flocks.

MARKETING SHEEP.

Until well on in the present century, the sheep trade of
the country was mainly conducted either privately on the
farms where the animals had been reared or fattened, or at
one or other of the fairs or markets held periodically in
various districts.

About forty years ago the first Live Stock Auction Mart
in Britain was opened by Messrs. A. Oliver & Son, Hawick.
The innovation was looked upon with suspicion at first; but
soon began to be regarded more favourably, and, once the
tide of public opinion turned, business increased with great
rapidity. The success which crowned the efforts of the
pioneers of the Auction movement led to the upspringing of
a host of imitators "here, there, and everywhere," and there
are now few towns, or even villages, of any size without
their Auctions.

As trade at these centres has increased, that at the farms
and markets has fallen off, and the drying-up process continues to extend with such rapidity that it seems probable
that ere long the whole of the sheep trade of the country
will be conducted through the medium of the Marts. Even
the old-established "Falkirk Tryst" itself seems likely to
to succumb. As an evidence of this, it may be mentioned
that at the October gathering last year the total number of
sheep exposed was only about 3000 ; whilst some of the old
frequenters of the Tryst present on that occasion, could
speak of seeing from 100,000 to 120,000 sheep on the ground.

The change is regarded by many as a great improvement
upon the old system, but by others it is looked upon as
not an unmixed blessing.

PREPARATIONS FOR SALE.

Passing, however, from the means of disposal, to the stock
to be disposed of, there are several matters—some of them at
first sight apparently of but little importance—attention to,
or neglect of, which, has a material effect in raising or lowering
the value of the sheep in the eyes of intending purchasers,
when they appear in the sale-ring.

In disposing of store sheep, the lot should be made as level
in every respect as possible, all inferior animals being drawn
out and sold by themselves. Some might be apt to think
that in a large lot the presence of a few inferior animals
would pass unnoticed, and that the price realized with these
included would be just as high as it would have been had
they been drawn out. This, however, is a mistake. There
is a class of buyers who will only purchase the best description of sheep, and another who deal mainly in secondary
lots. The latter rarely bid for superior lots, and the former
are generally chary in bidding when they observe that the
lot is wanting in uniformity.

In addition to drawing the sheep as equally as possible in regard to size, it is also important that they should resemble each other in the colour of the fleece, since, if some are of one shade and some of another, buyers may be apt to take them for a "made-up" lot, which, in their eyes would reduce their value.

To remedy this, it is customary in some quarters to pen the sheep pretty closely together a few days previous to sale, and shower over them water coloured by the addition of a small quantity of keel or ochre. A better plan, however, is to dip the sheep ten days or a fortnight before they are to be disposed of, taking care to employ a suitable dip ("*Cooper's*" *is the best*); this, in addition to rendering them all equal in colour, tends to open up the wool and make them look of greater size.

Fat sheep show to better advantage by having a little colour put on them—a slight touch of red keel on top of shoulder is amply sufficient.

Ordinary classes of "grit" ewes, and ewes with lambs at foot, are much improved in appearance by being 'carefully keeled.

The methods of preparing short-woolled and other breeds of sheep for show and sale are dealt with in another article. (*See Show Sheep.*)

LOADING SHEEP IN TRUCKS.

In forwarding sheep by rail the number placed in each truck should be regulated by various considerations apart from the size and condition of the animals. The length of the journey, season of the year, and purpose for which the sheep are intended when they reach their journey's end, should all be kept in mind.

During the winter season they may with safety be closer packed than in the summer time. If intended for sale immediately on landing at their destination it will be for their owner's interest to see that they are less closely packed than they might be if they were to have a week or two afterwards to recruit, before being disposed of. When crowded firmly together they lose "bloom" and appear dull and jaded-looking, which lessens their sale value.

Ewes and lambs should never be trucked together, unless there are very few of them. If a full load, the truck should be divided by hurdles—the ewes being placed at the one end and the lambs at the other. On an average about 40 clipped or 30 rough sheep, or 40 to 50 lambs may be taken as a fair load.

THE SHEPHERD'S CALENDAR.

It may here be desirable to gather up and tabulate some of the more important duties attaching to the farm, most of which are dealt with at greater length in other parts of the treatise.

Chronologists inform us that the Autumn season begins on 22nd September; Winter, 21st December; Spring, 20th March; and Summer on 21st June.

For our purpose we may regard the months of September, October, and November, as forming the Autumn quarter of the year—December. January, and February, the Winter—March, April, and May, the Spring—and June, July, and August, the Summer.

AUTUMN.

September.—Nature will now be showing symptoms of "the sere and yellow leaf," and, as the pastures will be failing, the condition of fattening sheep must be kept up by an increased supply of hand-feeding. The last sales of pure-bred rams are mostly held this month. It is essential that both ewes and rams should be in good condition previous to mating time. Hoggets and other sheep intended for winter feeding should be inured to their future rations by getting a few turnips daily spread and cut for them on the pasture. Weakly and poor-conditioned animals must be drawn out from the others, and have extra feeding given them, as, if allowed to fall into very poor order before commencing the box-feeding, there is frequently great difficulty in getting them to take to it. Cast ewes should now be got rid of. Sheep should never be allowed on wet land at this season of the year, as now and the succeeding month is the time when they lay the foundation of all parasitical diseases, Liver Fluke, Lung Worm, &c., &c. Rock Salt does more good now than at any other season.

October.—Wedders and other fattening sheep will now be settled down in their winter quarters, and should be liberally supplied with hay and box-feeding in addition to the roots. They should also have access to covered troughs containing rock-salt. Lambs should be provided with the best shelter possible, and have every reasonable care paid them, as this is their most critical period. This is the usual time for the disposal of cast ewes from hill farms. In purchasing such for crossing purposes, one should always endeavour to get them off *known* sound, healthy grazings. Although sheep from such "kent" places may sell at rather higher prices than others apparently as healthy, but from unknown quarters, it frequently happens that the dearest at the beginning are found the cheapest in the end. Bought-in sheep, whether for breeding or feeding, should be carefully dipped after being got home, as there is always a risk of scab breaking out amongst such new importations.

November.—The rams may now be removed from early served ewes, and the latter should be spread as thinly as possible over the pasture. All the sheep stock should be dipped this month, during favourable weather, to rid them of ticks and protect them during the winter months. See to all lame sheep, as foot-rot usually proves troublesome about this time. If any of the flock are affected with liver-rot, the disorder usually gives visible symptoms of its existence at this period of the year.

WINTER.

December.—Keep store and fattening sheep in a state of progressive improvement. Any standing still, in either class, means simply food thrown away. Sheep of every description, but especially hoggets confined on turnips, are now very liable to inflammatory attacks.

January.—See that during this, the coldest month of the year, the sheep are provided with the best possible shelter during stormy weather. The importance of warmth to all, but especially to breeding and fattening sheep, is indisputable. The animals will now in all probability be wholly dependent on hand-feeding; it is therefore important that regularity be observed 'n regard to their meal hours. Be very careful as to quality of food supplied to in-lamb ewes; particularly avoid giving them frosted turnips or over-abundance of any cold, succulent food.

February.—Avoid any sudden change in the feeding or other management of in-lamb ewes, as they will now be far advanced in pregnancy, and any such changes may lead to disastrous results. Provide comfortable shelter and all other things needful for the coming lambs. Don't put off such preparations till "the sweet by-and-bye," but "take time by the forelock." Hoggets will now be shedding their teeth; it is therefore essential that all turnips supplied to them be cut into finger-sized pieces, otherwise the animals may fall off seriously in condition.

SPRING.

March.—See remarks under last month. Shelter lambing ewes at night and also during daytime, unless the weather is moderately mild. If turnips are scarce and grass backward, supply them plentifully with box-feeding to keep up condition and promote flow of milk. Bear in mind that

> "If by halves you nourish the dams,
> You need only look for bad luck with the lambs."

With the first appearance of growth, "scour" is apt to prove troublesome amongst the sheep.

April.—See that the change from winter fare to the grass is not too abruptly brought about. A moderate allowance of bruised grain and bran for a few weeks at this period will tend to prevent excessive purging. Ewes and lambs should be carefully sheltered at night—at least in all exposed situations—in case of any sudden change taking place in the weather. Castrate lambs when about three weeks old, and dock them then or a week later. If moderately mild, fat sheep may be shorn previous to sale.

May.—In favourable situations hoggets may be shorn this month. It is, however, sometimes wise to defer clipping for a few weeks, since the old saying

> "Shear your sheep in May,
> Shear them all away,"

occasionally receives a partial fulfilment. If it is intended to wash the animals before clipping, the operation should be performed about eight or ten days previously.

SUMMER.

June.—This is the usual period for clipping. The sheep should be dipped about a month afterwards to rid them of vermin and protect from attacks of maggot-fly during the hot weather; for this purpose a poisonous dip is necessary. Ewes and lambs should undergo the operation at the same time, but separately. In wooded districts it is sometimes customary to smear the heads occasionally with a mixture of tar and brimstone. Cases of "hoove" are frequently met with at this season. We have entered more fully into dipping in another part of this work.

July.—Lambs may be weaned this month. In first placing them on aftermath, take advantage of dry weather for the purpose, as there is considerable risk of loss from hoove occurring if they are first placed on it when wet with dew or rain. The ewes should be placed on poor pasture until the milk dries off them, and all aged and faulty ones be afterwards drafted out for sale. Avoid disturbing the sheep during the heat of the day; all work amongst them should be done in the cool of the morning or evening.

August.—When early lambs are wanted, the rams may now be allowed out with the ewes. Be carefully on the outlook for maggot-struck sheep, especially if non-poisonous dips have been used in dipping. These are absolutely useless as preventives of such attacks. Weakly lambs, and other thin-conditioned animals, should, as a rule, be kept off the aftermath, and supplied with hand-feeding on the older pastures. It is in this month that the great sales of pure-bred rams are mostly held.

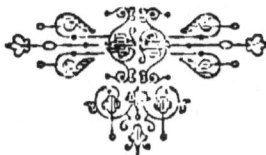

DISEASES OF SHEEP.

With regard to the diseases of sheep, although prevention is generally speaking easier than cure, and more economical, at the same time a knowledge of the general lines of treatment of the more common diseases to which sheep are liable is invaluable to the shepherd.

It is questionable whether any description of live stock have so little care bestowed on them—in so far as the attempt to treat in a satisfactory manner the disorders to which they are liable is concerned—as sheep; and this is the more to be regretted, as, owing to the weakness of their nervous system, the animals, if neglected in the earliest stage of attack, frequently fall victims to a disease which a little care and proper treatment on the first appearance of the trouble would have enabled them to throw off.

The old-fashioned method of slaughtering a sheep showing signs of illness, if in good condition, or of simply letting it take its chance, as is too often done, should it be poor, can hardly be considered altogether satisfactory. Were the symptoms shown at the onset of disease carefully noted and appropriate remedies then employed, the death rate in many flocks would be materially diminished.

The following are the most important medicines with which a shepherd should provide himself :—

Linseed, castor and olive oils, oil of turpentine, Epsom salts, laudanum, carbolic acid, sweet nitre, prepared chalk, carbonate of ammonia, ginger, gentian, catechu, and glycerine.

Caution is necessary in adapting the dose to the age and condition of the animal.

Of late years various firms have been selling medicine chests, containing preparations for the various disorders to which sheep are liable, and these chests have met with a considerable amount of favour, time and trouble being saved by having them at hand for any sudden emergency.

The administration of medicine to sheep.—The method recommended by the United States Department of Agriculture is as follows.—In giving medicine, drench from a horn, a spoon, or a stout glass bottle. Let an assistant throw the sheep on its haunches and hold it between his legs, back toward him—with the lower jaw seized in his left hand from the left side, he can either seize the upper jaw or pull out the cheek pouch with his right.

The following may be said to comprise most of the disorders to which sheep are liable :—

Abortion.
* Anthrax.
Aphtha Simple.
  do. Malignant.
Apoplexy.
Awalding or Rolling Over.
Black Leg.
Black Muzzle.
Bladder—Inflammation of.
Blindness or Optbalmia.
Braxy.
Broken Limbs.
Calculi.
Cancer.
Catarrh.
Colic.
Constipation.
Diarrhœa.
Downfall of Lamb Bed.
Dropping the Cud.
Dropsy.
Dysentry.
Eczema.
Fever in Lambs.
Fluke or Liver Rot.
* Foot and Mouth Disease.
Foot Rot.
Gad Fly.
Heaving or Straining.
Hoose or Husk.
Hoove.
Impaction of the Rumen.
  „   „   3rd Stomach.

Inflammation of the Lungs.
   „   „ Udder.
Jaundice or Yellows.
Joint-ill in Lambs.
Ked, commonly called Ticks.
Lice.
Liver Rot.
Lock Jaw.
Louping Ill.
Maggots.
Metritis, (Inflammation of the Womb.)
Nephritis, (Inflammation of the Kidneys.)
Opthalmia, (Inflammation of the Eyes.)
Paralysis.
Red Water.
Rickets.
Rupture.
* Scab.
Sore Eyes.
Sore Teats.
* Sheep Pox.
Sturdy.
Tape Worms.
The Tick.
Tuberculosis.
Tumours.
Water on the Brain.
Wool Balls in the Stomach.
Worms.
Wounds.

Those marked ° are subject to the provisions of the Contagious Diseases (Animals) Acts.

ABORTION—SLINKING, OR SLIPPING THE YOUNG.

The causes of this condition are excitement, crushing, over-driving, coming in contact with stakes or posts, &c., turning ewes for the purpose of dressing their feet when heavy in lamb, bad diet, eating ergotised or sewage grass, or an excessive amount of salt.

The symptoms are dulness, isolation from rest of the flock, with a discharge of a glairy fluid from the uterus, and upon a search being made the immature fœtus will probably be found in the pasture.

Treatment.—Remove the ewes which have aborted at once from the rest of the flock, protect them from cold, and inject a little carbolic oil into the genital passage (1 of carbolic acid to 30 of oil), and administer a dose of laxative medicine (3 oz. of castor oil combined with a drachm of laudanum.)

It is better to feed off animals that have aborted and not keep them round another year.

ANTHRAX.

This is a disease of an extremely fatal character, attacking animals upon certain pastures, and generally those which are in high condition and thriving rapidly. As a rule the sheep is found dead, the disease being of short duration :— The symptoms, if they should be observed, are great prostration with dulness, champing of the jaws, salivation, tremors, and sometimes, (if the animal lives long enough,) diarrhœa of a blood-stained colour. Death may be accompanied with convulsions, or the reverse. On post-mortem examination the spleen or melt is found greatly enlarged from engorgment by blood and sometimes the capsule is ruptured ; when cut across, the structure of the organ seems broken down and the contained blood is of a colour resembling damson jelly, staining the fingers. The bowels are sometimes greatly inflamed ; blood, similar in character to that found in the spleen, being thrown out between the coats thereof. The bladder may contain a quantity of chocolate-coloured urine. The veins underneath the skin are found to be full of black congealed blood; sometimes the lungs are highly congested, the blood being of the before-mentioned damson colour.

Extreme care should be exercised in opening the carcase of an animal which has died showing symptoms of anthrax, as the slightest abrasion on the hands or arms of the operator may lead to fatal results from blood poisoning. Before commencing the operation a solution of one part of carbolic acid and fifteen parts of oil or glycerine should be smeared over the hands.

The disease is spread by means of rod-shaped bacilli (*bacillus anthracis*). These generate with great rapidity in the blood stream of the living animal. They have also the peculiar characteristic, when brought into contact with the oxygen of the atmosphere, of changing into spores. These become covered with a thick coating which protects them from heat and cold and other influences that otherwise would destroy their vitality. They may thus remain dormant in the pasture or elsewhere for an incredibly long period, resuming their previous condition, and setting up the disease in a healthy animal as soon as they are again taken into the system. This accounts for the extreme difficulty of cleansing a pasture which has once been infected from a case of anthrax, a condition of things that becomes aggravated where a diseased sheep has been buried in the field, unless deeply covered and disinfected, as these spores may be brought to the surface with the casts of the earth worm at any time.

Treatment of affected animals is of no avail. Carcases should be buried 6-ft. deep in some spot over which sheep are not likely to graze, and well covered with quick lime,

care being taken that they are not placed where there is
danger of contaminating the water courses. Where possible,
burning is the most effectual way of disposing of the carcase; neither the wool nor the skin should be made use
of. The pasture should be dug up spade deep from the
spot where the animal was found dead, and thoroughly
burned, or mixed with quick lime. The remaining sheep
should, if possible, be removed to another pasture, or if
this cannot be done, change their food entirely, and give
a dose of salts (3 oz.); see that they are well supplied with
salt, and administer once a day chlorate of potash in 20
grain doses in water, or mixed with the food.

On the Continent vaccination has been largely resorted to
as a preventive, and is claimed to have produced excellent
results, but the question cannot yet be considered as settled.

APHTHA (SIMPLE,) OR THRUSH IN THE MOUTH.

This disease is most common in lambs, though sometimes
it affects older sheep. In the latter it is said to be due to
irritant vegetable matters, or to stomach irregularities. In
the former it arises from derangement of the system of
the ewe.

Symptoms—salivation, smacking of the mouth, and disinclination to eat. On examining the mouth the lining
membrane is found to be in a bare and ulcerated condition
with redness and swelling of the underlying tissues. The
bowels are irregular and frequently relaxed.

Treatment.—In lambs, change the mother's diet and give
about thirty grains of salt petre daily in their food; apply to
the sores a saturated solution of alum, to which a little borax
and glycerine have been added. To older animals give a dose
of laxative medicine, change the food, dress the mouth with
the above-mentioned solution, and protect them from cold
and wet.

APHTHA (MALIGNANT)

arises from blood derangement of the ewe, manifested by the presence of sores on the teats and thighs. These sores are of an infective nature, causing similar sores on portions of the body with which they may come in contact. Lambs sucking from teats so affected show severe ulceration of the lips and gums, the latter sometimes becoming so deeply involved that the teeth become loose and fall out. The lambs lose condition rapidly, and may die from diarrhœa and exhaustion.

Treatment.—Change the pasture, shelter the ewes, feed well, give a dram of hyposulphite of soda twice a day (sprinkled in the food if they will eat it), draw off the milk and dress the sores with a watery solution of carbolic acid, 1 part acid, 20 parts water, and adding to this as much alum as it will take up. The lambs must be artificially fed if necessary, and the sores in the mouth touched first with a solution of perchloride of iron and then treated as in the case of simple aphtha.

APOPLEXY.

Under the head of "Braxy" will be found as much information of this disease as the farmer is likely to require.

AWALDING OR ROLLING OVER.

This, though not strictly speaking a disease, occasions more loss to the farmer than anything else, indeed, in many flocks, more than all his misfortunes combined.

With the advent of the warm season, sheep, previous to being shorn, are frequently a source of trouble and anxiety to the shepherd, owing to the habit some of them have of rolling over on their backs, and being unable to rise without assistance. Ewes are often troublesome in this manner when near lambing, and if not quickly relieved from their awkward position die in a very short time. Awalding is in most cases

due to the presence of ticks on the skin, and dipping in the
autumn and spring months is the best preventive.

BLACK LEG OR BLACK QUARTER.

A disease identical with that affecting cattle but not so
common. The affected animal ceases to eat, isolates itself,
is disinclined to move, parts of the body become swollen, and
if the disease should locate itself in the limbs the animal is
extremely lame. Sometimes a side is affected, sometimes the
head and neck, and sometimes the hind quarters; in sheep,
more frequently than cattle, the swelling is disposed to spread,
the tissues rapidly undergoing a state of decomposition. The
swelling is at first hot and tender, but rapidly becomes cold,
insensible, charged with gas, and upon pressure imparts a
crackling sensation to the fingers. Death usually occurs in
the course of a few hours.

Treatment of those affected is practically useless, but preventive measures should be taken with regard to the unaffected; if possible change the pasture, but at any rate
change the food, and ensure the animals taking a certain
amount of exercise. Dose with hyposulphite of soda or
sulphate of iron, one drachm of either to each sheep, in
water, or with the food in the feeding troughs.

BLACK MUZZLE.

This term has been applied to a scabby eruption sometimes
occurring on the nose and lips of sheep, and which is
attributed to the presence of some noxious plants in the
pasture. A rapid cure can be effected by rubbing well daily
with ointment composed of 1 oz. powdered burnt alum, 1 oz.
powdered zinc sulphate, and 12 oz. lard.

BLADDER—INFLAMMATION OF.

This disease is rarely met with save amongst rams and
then it is usually associated with calculi or stone, which will
be dealt with elsewhere. The symptoms are described under

the heading "Calculi," and are in both cases alike. When the two are associated the urine is passed very frequently and in small quantities, with great pain.

Treatment.—Withhold corn and roots and give good hay with plenty of linseed gruel. Administer a mild purgative and give twice daily, one drachm tincture of opium, and two drachms sweet spirits nitre.

BLINDNESS (SEE OPTHALMIA.)

BRAXY.

This is seen in sheep rapidly thriving, and receiving a very liberal allowance of swede turnips and highly nutritious food. The animals suddenly fall down dead from violent congestion of the brain or apoplexy—some such cases may be anthrax. Slaughter immediately if seen before dead, as the carcase may be unaffected.

Prevention.—Stop giving corn for a few days, and administer to each sheep a mild dose of aperient medicine such as salts, 2 to 3 ounces, with a little ginger, and let the sheep have more exercise by running on to a bare pasture for a few hours daily. Allow plenty of salt with food, and give occasional doses of saltpetre.

BROKEN LIMBS.

Sheep suffering from broken limbs—generally resulting from their getting entangled in wire-fences, and similar causes—should be confined in a shed or yard till recovery. Place the broken bones in proper position as quickly as possible after the accident, and tightly splinter the limb—a piece of soft leather being wound firmly round *under* the splints, which are best secured by a strong linen bandage soaked in starch. The bandages may in most cases be removed in the course of three weeks and a plain dry bandage put on.

CALCULI OR STONES.

These are by no means rare in sheep, and are classified according to the situations they are met with in the urinary apparatus.

Any portion of the urinary canal is liable to these deposits, which result from the urine containing excess of salts in solution, liberated from the blood in the kidneys.

When present in the kidneys they are termed renal calculi, containing large quantities of Lime salts; cystic and urethral calculi, when in the bladder and urethral canal in which the triple phosphate of ammonia and magnesia is in excess; and preputial calculi when abundant around the sheath or wool at the opening of the urinary passage.

Causes—which tend to produce this condition in either sex are those of forced feeding on highly nitrogenous foods, such as beans, peas, corn with mangolds, &c., and usually accompanied with too little exercise.

The phosphates in the grain accumulate, and urea results in too large quantities from the decomposition of the nitrogenous principles.

The urine becomes acid instead of alkaline due to the presence of uric and silicic acids, which, when liberated from the blood through the kidneys along the bladder or urethral canal, have a tendency to become deposited.

In the male, the worm of the penis is very much contracted, and the flow of urine is somewhat small. It is not an uncommon occurrence to find numbers of small calculi hanging from the wool and hair at the end of the sheath, where they have become deposited from the constant trickling down of the urine saturated with the materials in solution.

Symptoms.—Refusal of food, panting, grunting, colicky pains, constant straining, general restlessness, bad cases unable to rise, and, unless relieved, death results from absorption of urine into the system, (uræmia.)

Treatment.—Examine the urinary passage, if calculi are found adhering to the sheath or wool of the belly, wash thoroughly, and dress with carbolic oil, clip off all wool, and administer internally 8 to 16 grains of extract of belladonna, followed by a dose of opening medicine.

Removal of the cause in so far as is practicable, lessening the liability of the rest of the flock to this condition, and the fact that sheep out at grass do not suffer from this condition indicates that flocks liable to this disorder should be turned out on pasture and fed low.

In some cases the calculus, if felt, is cut down on with a sharp knife and enucleated, or, if confined to the worm, this has to be excised to allow the escape of the deposit.

If any treatment is not practicable have the animal slaughtered at once before fever or uræmia set in.

N.B.—Cases described as "red water" are probably conditions arising from the colouring of the urine red from a highly nitrogenous food, as we have no evidence that the disease spoken of as "red water" in cattle has an analogy in sheep.

CANCER.

When this occurs dispose of the animal to the butcher at the most favorable opportunity.

CATARRH.

The symptoms of this disorder, usually arising from long-continued exposure to cold and wet, are a cough, running of water from the eyes, mucous discharge from the nostrils, dulness, and in severe cases, loss of appetite. The necessary treatment consists in keeping the animals comfortably sheltered, feeding well, and giving daily in a little linseed tea (until they are fairly on the road to recovery), 1 drachm sweet spirits of nitre, and 15 grains powdered digitalis.

COLIC.

The symptoms are those of acute pain of an intermittent nature, usually caused by over-feeding on new succulent pasture, or drinking cold water after being heated by driving.

The most successful treatment consists in giving, in a little warm gruel, 1 drachm landanum, 1 drachm powdered ginger, and 3 or 4 ozs. sulphate of magnesia—repeating in the course of two hours if necessary, omitting the magnesia.

CONSTIPATION.

Constipation of the bowels is in great measure, if not wholly, due to the pasture or food being of too dry and binding a nature. Purgatives should be freely administered to open the bowels, and the animals removed to more succulent pasture.

In cases where young lambs are affected the trouble is generally due to some defect in the quality of the milk given by the ewe. An entire change of food should therefore be given to the latter, and a teaspoonful of castor-oil to the lamb daily, and injections of tepid water into the rectum till there are signs of improvement.

DIARRHŒA.

This trouble, more frequently termed " scour," is most common amongst young sheep, and usually caused by derangement of the stomachs and bowels by irritant or indigestible food, or from diet being too rich and plentiful. It is, as a rule, most prevalent during wet weather, and when hoar frost prevails. The ailing sheep should be placed on less succulent food, and have a tablespoonful of castor oil given (in order to clear the intestines ;) and twice a day afterwards, till there are signs of improvement, give two tablespoonfuls of the following mixture :—Powdered ginger, 4 drachms ; catechu, 4 drachms ; opium, ½ drachm ; prepared chalk, 12 drachms ; peppermint water, ½ pint. Shake the bottle well before use.

Lambs are occasionally attacked by a very dangerous form of diarrhœa, termed, from the colour of the fæces, *White Scour*. This trouble is due to coagulation of the milk in the fourth stomach by the action of rennett separating it into curds and whey; the former undergoes coagulation and blocks up the passage, the whey alone passing off by the bowels. The malady usually attacks lambs when only a few days old, and frequently proves fatal.

Treatment.—Allow the lamb to take but little or no milk from the ewe until on the way to recovery, but give frequently instead, a little well-cooked linseed gruel with a small quantity of brandy in it. No medicine can be better than that recommended above for older sheep, but of course it must be given in much smaller quantities according to the size of the lamb.

DOWNFALL OF LAMB-BED.

Inversion of the womb, or downfall of the lamb-bed, is of somewhat common occurrence after severe cases of lambing, and even occurs occasionally when the ewes lamb quite easily and without assistance. To replace it, turn the ewe on her back, with the hind-quarters raised well up, and, after anointing the hands with carbolic oil, bathe the womb with lukewarm water, by means of a sponge, to cleanse it from any dirt adhering to it. Replace it in its natural position by gently pressing it back, but taking care not to injure it. Confine it in its place by means of one or two stitches passed through the lips of the external parts. Should the womb have been exposed for a time, however, and become swollen and inflamed, it is scarcely possible to keep it retained, as the ewe is apt to press so violently as to burst the sutures through the lips of the orifice. In such cases 2 or 3 drachms of laudanum should be given in gruel, and a little carbolic solution (1 part acid to 20 parts olive oil) injected into the

womb, and the hind parts still raised up. This treatment
may ease the ewe and cause her to cease paining.

DROPPING THE CUD.

Indigestion is generally the cause of this trouble, which in
every case is marked by the dribbling of saliva from the
mouth.

The treatment necessary to effect a cure consists in administering a purgative—such as Epsom salts, and giving the
animal an entire change of food. The free use of salt acts as
a preventative.

In some cases it arises from a displaced tooth, or some
foreign substance getting fixed in the mouth. A close examination should therefore always be made, and, if found,
the offending substance removed.

DROPSY (SANGUINEOUS ASCITES).

Is seen generally in sheep which have been exposed to
inclement weather, (particularly cold and wet combined,)
badly fed, and insufficiently sheltered. The use of rotten
turnips is an especial cause.

Symptoms—resemble somewhat those of advanced liver-
rot, the eyes are bloodless and watery looking, a dropsical
swelling appears beneath the jaw, and the belly is distended
sometimes enormously, there is disinclination to move, excessive panting if exerted. The urine may be voided frequently in large quantity and of a pale colour. The bowels
are constipated at first then relaxed. In extreme cases no
urine may be passed at all ; here the diarrhœa is still more
marked and death follows shortly. The carcase on examination is found to be dropsical, the flesh is pale and watery,
and the fluid is thrown out into the body cavities, the kidneys
are generally soft and pulpy resembling in consistence a
rotten pear. For sheep thus affected little can be done,
proper shelter combined with generous feeding, and the

administration of tonics, as sulphate of iron 1 scruple and
gentian 2 drachms, daily, may bring some of them round,
but though many of them linger for considerable periods
they seldom do much good. Prevention in subsequent
seasons by drainage of land, better feeding, and improved
shelter are advisable.

DYSENTRY

Is an aggravated form of Diarrhœa and requires more urgent
treatment. The medicine recommended for Diarrhœa is the
best that can be adopted, but should be given in larger doses
and the quantity of brandy increased.

In very bad cases an enema of gruel and laudanum should
be given to allay the inflammation.

ECZEMA.

A skin disease affecting the face and legs of sheep browsing on luxuriant pastures, (particularly those containing
alsike clover in flower,) or sheep turned out on sandy pastures.
Where animals are exposed to cold blasts of rain, the back
and sides are the seat of the disease. The skin of the affected
parts become swollen, hot, and tender, crops of vesicles appear; these burst and scabs are formed which are sometimes
mistaken for "scab" proper. The two are, however, easily
distinguished. In eczema the sheep manifest pain when
scratched instead of evincing pleasure, moreover the scabs
are not so distinct nor so extensive as in "scab," and the
parasite is absent.

Treatment.—Remove to other pastures if possible. Smear
the lips, when these are affected, with an ointment composed
of one part of boracic acid to six or eight of lard or vaseline.
To the limbs and back, applications of an astringent lotion
of alum, glycerine, and water answers very well.

FEVER IN LAMBS.

The symptoms present in this disorder are rapid loss of

condition, severe diarrhœa, and troublesome cough when disturbed. In many cases the trouble is due to the presence of parasites in the lungs, (see *Hoose*). In others, to exposure during long-continued cold and wet weather.

Ailing lambs should be liberally supplied with nourishing food, or gruel if the appetite is impaired, and sheltered at night. A teaspoonful of turpentine (or less if the patient is very young) may be given in half a wine-glass of linseed oil, and repeated two or three times at intervals of two days. One drachm nitrate of potass and 12 grains emetic tartar in linseed gruel, may also with benefit be administered twice a day for a few days.

FLUKE (SEE LIVER ROT.)

FOOT AND MOUTH DISEASE.

This disease is identical with that in cattle, and the infection may be conveyed from the one to the other. It usually lasts from ten days to three weeks.

Symptoms.—Sudden lameness, dulness, isolation, shivering, perhaps coughing, and sometimes slight diarrhœa. In the feet the eruption usually shows itself around the coronet, in front of each digit, and at the heel, and not rarely around the supernumerary digits. In appearance it somewhat resembles a bleb, or blister. On breaking this a watery fluid exudes, and a very raw, red surface is left exposed, which becomes covered in the course of two or three days with a brownish scab. In severe cases the vesicles may extend right round the coronet, and when such sheep are travelled, casting of one hoof is not uncommon. Some authorities consider mouth lesions rare in sheep. When they are present they are small and confined to the lips and pad. In pregnant ewes abortion very often occurs. The disease is generally met with in a mild form, but should it assume a malignant character the animals affected waste rapidly, the fever remains high, and death from exhaustion follows.

Treatment.—Protect from the weather. Isolate diseased from healthy animals. If the sheep are grazing, cut grass for them, otherwise provide them with succulent food. Give saline medicine such as hyposulphite of soda in doses of 1 or 2 drachms daily, or chlorate of potash in half drachm doses. Apply to the sores on the feet a wash of 10 parts carbolic acid and 10 of alum to 100 parts of water, this may be placed in a shallow trough, hurdled on each side, and the sheep walked through it 3 or 4 times. During recovery small doses of gentian and iron (one drachm of gentian to half a drachm of iron) are beneficial. As a rule, no great amount of treatment is bestowed upon this disease. Sheep which have been affected, and those in contact with them, should be isolated from healthy flocks for at least three weeks.

FOOT ROT.

This troublesome disorder prevails to a greater or less extent on all lands, but especially on rich low-lying pastures, and is usually most prevalent during the autumn months, when the ground is wet from heavy dews and rains. Unfortunately it is so common that every sheepowner is too well acquainted with the symptoms for it to be necessary to give them here.

Treatment.—Remove all loosened and diseased portions of the horn, and shorten long feet, with a very sharp knife, but care should be taken not to cut deep enough to make the feet bleed, as that is injurious. Many kinds of specifics are in use, and generally speaking, some of these may be procured from chemists; this saves all trouble of mixing. Butter of antimony and tincture of myrrh in equal parts is a very good dressing, so is an ointment composed of one ounce finely powdered sulphate copper to 6 or 8 ounces of lard, to which, after well rubbing down, one drachm of finely powdered corrosive sublimate is added. Where flocks are large it is found advantageous to drive the sheep through a trough containing a mixture of Cooper's Dip, one packet to a gallon of water. This should simply be deep enough to cover the hoofs, and after being driven through, the sheep should be penned on a bare spot for a few hours afterwards. Many authorities consider foot rot contagious, especially that form commencing between the digits, hence it is advisable to separate the healthy from the affected animals and put the latter on a dry, well drained pasture.

GAD FLY.

The proper name for this fly is *Oestrus Ovis*. It deposits its eggs on the edge of the nostrils of the sheep, and the larvæ find their way into the nasal passages and the sinuses of the head of the sheep, giving rise to severe catarrhal symptoms, and causing what is popularly known as "grub in the head." The fly somewhat resembles a small brown bee. They usually appear in June and July, and the length of time the larvæ take to pass through their full development in the nasal chambers is about 10 months. Sheep manifest great excitement when attacked by the fly, huddling together in some dry, dusty spot, with their noses close to the ground. As the larvæ mature they work their way upwards into the head by means of their hooks and spines. There is a profuse flow of mucus from the affected nostril, with frequent sneezing. Sometimes the animals suffer from attacks of giddiness, and even death ensues. The mature larvæ is about $\frac{3}{4}$ of an inch long. When small they are white; as they increase in size they become yellow, with a black band running along the back. When fully grown they move back towards the nostrils and are expelled in the act of sneezing, fall to the ground and pass through a pupa stage before appearing as flies, between April and end of July.

Treatment—which is not very satisfactory—consists in the injection into the nasal cavities of some agent destructive to the parasite. This may be done as follows :—Procure an elastic bulb syringe with a small nozzle about 6 inches long, and practice with it a few times until able to expel about a teaspoonful at a time. Fill the syringe with olive oil and turpentine in equal quantities, pass the nozzle of the syringe up the nostril, and by a sharp movement inject about a teaspoonful; withdraw the syringe and in a few moments serve the other nostril in the same manner.

Prevention.—A means of prevention is to apply to the noses of the sheep with a brush a mixture of equal parts of tar and whale or fish oil once every two or three days during the hot summer weather. Or the following ointment may be used in the same way :—Beeswax, 1 lb. ; linseed oil, 1 pint ; melt together with two ounces common resin, and, as this cools, stir in 4 ounces of carbolic acid.

HEAVING, OR STRAINING,

which usually terminates in inflammation of the womb. The trouble is in most cases due either to the ewes being in too high condition, or to some injury inflicted whilst giving assistance in lambing. Some consider it infectious.

In any case in which there has been difficulty in lambing, it is a mistaken policy to wait until disease manifests itself before adopting treatment. The endeavour should be to prevent trouble arising, rather than trusting to remedial measures after it appears. As a preventive, a little gruel containing 2 drachms laudanum and 2 oz. linseed or castor oil should be given, and a little carbolic solution—1 part acid to 40 parts olive oil—injected into the womb.

If heaving arises, 3 drachms of laudanum should be given, and repeated a few hours after, if needful, and a stronger carbolic solution (1 part acid to 20 parts oil) employed. An

animal suffering from heaving should be put right away
from other ewes, and some one instead of the shepherd
should attend her, otherwise it may extend to other members
of the flock.

HOOSE OR HUSK

or parasitic bronchitis is a form of lung disease arising
from the presence in the lungs and air passages of the sheep,
of a delicate white worm 1½ to 2 inches long, *(strongylus
filaria.)* The disease is most common towards the end of
summer and in autumn, particularly when the weather is
warm and moist, as these conditions seem favourable to a
prolonged existence of the parasite outside the body of its
host. It mostly attacks young animals up to two years old.

Symptoms.—Difficulty in breathing, particularly if hurried,
when they manifest discomfort by repeated husky coughing
and sometimes expel the worms in the act; the skin and
wool are dry, and the mucous membranes bloodless. In
severe cases these conditions are so marked as to give rise to
the term " paper skin." As the disease progresses the coughing becomes more frequent and exhausting, and death results
either from the disease produced in the lungs or from
exhaustion arising from the diarrhœa, which accompanies the
later stages. On opening the air passages of the lungs after
death, numbers of the filaria are found, so there is no difficulty
in detecting the cause of death. Old pastures which have
not been turned up for many years are the most dangerous,
though the disease is said to have occurred on second year's
clover. The eggs of the filaria pass their early life in the
body of the common earth worm. They are brought to the
surface in the casts and contaminate the pastures. Having
gained entrance per the digestive system in the blood, they
are quickly carried to the lungs, where they mature, and the
irritation they set up in the bronchial tubes, causes coughing

when the embryos are deposited on the pasture, thus affecting healthy sheep.

Treatment.—In its early stage the disease is amenable to treatment. Several methods find favour, the most simple being the administration, every second day for a week, of equal quantities of turpentine and linseed oil in tablespoonful doses, with such a tonic as gentian.

Inhalation of gas, (chlorine or sulphur fumes) is frequently very effectual. The sheep are driven into a close shed, the doors and windows of which are carefully stopped up, and the gas is liberated, in the case of chlorine by pouring sulphuric acid in a mixture of manganese di-oxide and common salt, or in the case of sulphur fumes by placing powdered sulphur on a red hot shovel, or over a charcoal fire, or by igniting cones made of a mixture of sulphur and charcoal to which sufficient gum arabic has been added, to give consistence. The duration and intensity of the fumigation should be regulated according to the tolerance of the sheep, and it is as well that someone should remain in the place with them to see that none are overcome. Should such a thing happen the animal should be at once removed into the open air. Two or three fumigations frequently suffice. A more scientific and effectual method than either of these has lately been introduced, that of injecting into the windpipe, by means of a syringe armed with a hollow sharp-pointed needle, a quantity of medicine which rapidly volatilises when in contact with the lung tissue, and acting directly on the parasites kills them. The following mixture is suitable,—ten minims of medicinal carbolic acid, fifteen minims of chloroform, and thirty minims of turpentine. The method of administration is as follows:—the animal's neck is put on the stretch, by elevating the nose, the needle of the syringe is introduced into the windpipe between the rings about half way down the neck, and the medicine is forced drop by drop into it slowly, or violent coughing ensues. Two or three such doses at intervals of two days are usually effectual, excepting, of course, in cases too advanced to admit of any treatment.

Preventive measures.—Plough up and lime affected pastures, if possible. Failing this, keep sheep off them for a year or two, and do not even then overcrowd them; drain the pastures, keep the sheep from all swampy parts, and if they drink from a running stream it should be fenced off except at the point where they drink. Give a liberal quantity of dry nourishing food, and supply them with salt. Affected animals should be kept from the healthy, and carefully protected from the weather.

HOOVE OR HOVEN.

A condition in which the rumen or first stomach becomes distended with gas, the result of fermentation of its contents, seen when sheep are feeding on succulent food such as clover, or after browsing on grass heavily laden with dew, or covered with hoar frost, or on frosted roots.

Symptoms—dulness, hurried breathing, and distension of the abdomen, particularly on the left side.

Treatment.—When interference with respiration is extreme the rumen should be tapped on the left side with a trocar and cannula at its most prominent point, and the gas allowed to escape. In less urgent cases the administration of a dose of spirits of ammonia 3 to 4 drachms, hypo-sulphite soda 1 drachm with a drachm of ginger, in half a pint of cold water every four hours, followed shortly by a purgative dose of Epsom salts combined with ginger, will suffice. Care should be exercised in feeding, and excess of succulent materials should be avoided.

IMPACTION OF THE RUMEN OR PLEXALVIAS.

A similar condition of the rumen, from distension with food may be noticed here; this is often due to excess of dry unnutritious food, to animals eating the coarse withered herbage so commonly seen in late autumn, and to sudden alterations of dieting from indifferent food, to palatable and nutritious food given in excess. The animals are dull, refuse to eat, the bowels are constipated, breathing is difficult, and the distended abdomen, instead of feeling tympanitic as in the last case, has a doughy feel, though a certain amount of gas may be present.

Treatment.—Give purgative with ginger as in the last case. In extreme cases the organ is sometimes opened through the flank, and about two-thirds of its contents removed, but this requires skill, and at the best is dangerous. Feed carefully for some time after recovery.

IMPACTION OF THE THIRD STOMACH, OR GRASS STAGGERS,

or "fardel bound," may occur from similar causes to the last. Here the animal is likely to show more pain. In the early stages there is apparent diarrhœa, followed by constipation. Liberal doses of castor or linseed oils are serviceable, but should they fail, a good dose of salts and ginger, combined with eight grains of powdered nux vomica, repeated again in ten or twelve hours generally answers well.

INFLAMMATION OF THE LUNGS (PNEUMONIA).

This disease, arising from exposure to cold and wet, is seldom met with amongst sheep; but cases are sometimes experienced, should inclement weather prevail shortly after shearing, and in show animals on exposure to cold in travelling from a confined, and usually heated atmosphere. The chief symptoms are, (1) rapid breathings and failure of strength, (2) feverishness, painful cough. The patient must be kept warm, and the following mixture given in a little

linseed tea :—2 drachms sweet spirits of nitre, 2 tablespoonfuls of whiskey or gin. Repeat in six hours if not better.

INFLAMMATION OF THE UDDER (MAMMITIS).

This disorder (occasionally termed *garget*) is frequently
met with in ewes, shortly after lambing, or after lambs have
been taken away, and as a rule is most prevalent during cold
stormy weather. Sometimes it arises from sore teats.
Attention is usually first drawn to the matter by the thin
appearance of the lamb and the evident disinclination of the
ewe to allow the lamb to suck, or by the ewe walking with
hind legs wide apart. On examination the udder is found
swollen, painful, and inflamed. Ewes suffering in this way
should be confined in warm quarters till recovery, as exposure to cold favours the progress of the malady.

Treatment.—Give purgative. In mild cases the lamb
should be kept to the ewe four or five times daily to remove
the milk, the udder frequently fomented with warm water,
and afterwards well rubbed with a mixture of turpentine
1 ounce, and olive oil 10 ounces, twice a day ; or with belladonna ointment made with lard in the proportions of 1 to 8.

In severe cases it may be necessary to remove the lamb
and draw off the milk or watery secretion by hand. Treat
as above. Should abscesses form, open when ready by
means of a lancet and apply a linseed-meal poultice, afterwards bathing frequently with a weak solution of carbolic
acid in water or oil.

JAUNDICE, OR YELLOWS.

The visible symptoms in this disorder are a yellow appearance of the skin and mucous membrane, due to an interference
with the secretion of bile from the liver, and re-absorption
into the blood, accompanied by irregular appetite, and
costiveness of the bowels, the urine being of a dark brown
colour. Sheep pasturing on rich grass are most frequently

affected. The liberal use of salt is the best preventive. Ailing animals should have an entire change of food, and the bowels be freely moved by the aid of Epsom salts—2 to 4 ounces, according to age and size, or calomel 10 grains in gruel, and repeated after an interval of two or three days if necessary.

JOINT-ILL IN LAMBS.

This is a trouble regarding which changeable weather has much to do, and as it is more common on some farms than on others, it may be that it is due to some peculiarity in the soil, or to the management. Lambs reared in cold, wet, exposed districts are most frequently affected.

The symptoms somewhat resemble those of rheumatism, but sometimes abscesses form in the joints and discharge their contents, leaving open joints. The animals attacked should be kept well sheltered, and treated kindly by giving stimulants and tonics in gruel. This disease, like many others, is easier prevented than cured. To prevent it, keep on dry pasture and afford good shelter.

THE KED—COMMONLY CALLED TICK,

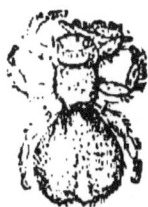

or *Melophagus Ovinus*, is frequently confounded with the true tick, to which, however, it has not the slightest resemblance. The eggs of the former are in shape and color like the pippin of an apple, and are attached to the wool by a sticky substance secreted from the female.

These insect pests, which propagate with great rapidity, have a very hurtful effect on sheep—keeping the animals in a state of constant irritation and restlessness, and causing them to go off their feed and lose condition. They are seen nibbling at their sides, rolling on their backs, or rubbing against fences to relieve the intense itching of the skin due to the keds moving about and the poison they exude while feeding. In this way the fleece is broken and much loss of wool arises, while in the spring with a heavy fleece many sheep may die through awalding.

The insects pass readily from sheep to sheep, and in warm weather can live on the pasture a considerable time. Thorough dipping *with a poisonous dip* is the only method of effectually exterminating them and of keeping the fleece from further attack, as *non-poisonous dips* only kill the living keds, leaving the eggs to hatch and thrive, and in a short time the evil is as great as ever.

LICE.

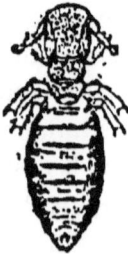

The true louse of the sheep *(Trichodectes Sphærocephalus)* is a minute red-headed insect about one-twenty-fifth of an inch long, very seldom seen in England. It is most numerous in those parts of the body poorly protected by wool, as between the legs and body. It is most common in young animals and has a very deleterious effect on the quantity and quality of the wool, and makes the animals restless and uneasy so that they cannot thrive. The ked is sometimes wrongly classed with the louse family.

Treatment.—These pests are destroyed by dipping.

LIVER ROT.

This deadly disease, the most serious with which the flockmaster has to contend, is due to the presence of the mature form of the liver fluke, *(distoma hepaticum)* in the liver and bile passages. In some marshy, low lying, and ill drained farms this is a perfect scourge to sheep-owners, causing enormous losses. The adult fluke is from three-quarters of an inch to an inch in length, flattened and brownish in colour, and from one-eighth to half-an-inch broad. It inhabits the bile passages of the liver, deriving its nourishment from the

blood of its host, and causing by its presence a chronic inflammation, which alters the liver structure so as to deprive
it of its proper function. The eggs are expelled into the bile
ducts, thence into the intestines, and are ejected with the
droppings; should they reach water, they are hatched, the
embryos swimming about by means of delicate hair-like
processes till they encounter their next host, a small snail *(the
Limnæus Truncatulatus,)* about one-third of an inch long.
They burrow into its body, and there undergo two further
transformations, escaping once more in a fourth form into
the water. This fourth form, which differs widely from the
adult fluke, adheres to the leaves of grasses and water plants,
and is picked up by sheep and cattle while grazing. They
thus enter the digestive system, finding their way into the
liver, and there develope into the mature fluke. At first
they are small, and cause but little inconvenience. As they
grow, the irritation they set up causes an increased flow of
bile, and for a time the sheep fatten with a rapidity which
experienced sheep-owners look upon as extremely suspicious.
The mucous membranes of the eye, etc., at the first part of
this stage are somewhat pale, and become yellow towards its
termination. About three months after infection the sheep
enter upon another stage—the yellow mucous membranes
become blanched, the eyes watery looking; the animals are
listless, the wool harsh, dry, and falling off. Abortion occurs
among the ewes; dropsical swellings appear under the jaws,
and fœtid diarrhœa sets in. Animals most frequently die in
this stage which lasts about three weeks; should the animal
last over this, it may to a certain extent rally, but rarely, if
ever, becomes restored to a state of health. The liver, when
examined in advanced cases, seems of a blueish colour with
white bands running across it. It cuts firmly and often
grates on the knife. The bile ducts are thickened, and in

their interior the mature flukes, along with a quantity of olive green material, are found.

The disease is difficult to eradicate, but drainage, fencing off swampy places, and the application of salt or lime, 5 cwt. to the acre during the first part of June, July, and August, is generally beneficial. Manure of rotten sheep should be mixed with lime, and should not be placed on moist ground. Diseased livers should be burned. Do not overstock the pastures, as the more sheep there are, the closer they will graze, and the more likely they are to pick up the infected grasses. If sheep are grazed on ground known to be infested they should have a daily allowance of salt and dry food. For convalescent sheep, sulphate of iron and salt mixed with the food are the most effectual tonics, 15 to 20 grains sulphate of iron, with a teaspoonful of salt, daily for each sheep.

Administration of medicine for the cure of the disease when it is established is of little use.

LOCK-JAW.

This trouble occasionally results from exposure to cold and wet, but is more frequently due to some injury—such as exposure after shearing, castrating, or docking. The animal attacked should be kept very warm. Castor oil should be administered, followed by 2 to 4 drachms of laudanum and the same quantity of powdered ginger in a little warm gruel. The patient should be as little disturbed as possible, as quietude seems to be of vital importance in such cases. Better slaughter the animal if in good condition than attempt treatment.

LOUPING-ILL.

Various theories have been promulgated as to the cause of this nervous disorder, which is somewhat common during the spring months, particularly during long-continued wet weather, and on farms exposed to the cold easterly winds usually prevalent at that season of the year. It seems only reasonable to conclude that the disorder is actually due to these hurtful influences.

The symptoms vary considerably in different cases. Most usually the animal is seized with trembling fits, loses the power of its legs, and lies on its side, grinding its teeth and moving its limbs convulsively—lingering possibly for days till death ends its sufferings.

The use of strong purgatives is said to have occasionally led to a cure ; but to be of service the treatment must be adopted on the first symptoms of the trouble being visible.

Shelter, during inclement weather, may be regarded as the best preventive, and here again prevention is better than cure.

MAGGOTS.

It is probable that this pest is more prevalent and makes greater demands upon the shepherd than all the other ailments of the flock combined. It is caused by the larvæ of the common blow-fly or flesh-fly, which in the summer months, particularly in warm showery weather, and in low lying or woody districts, deposits its eggs on sores or on damp or dirty wool so generally found on the hind parts of the sheep. These become hatched into grubs, which quickly work their way into the skin, causing fearful torture, and if neglected, the death of the sheep. The suffering animal has a restless or excitable manner, with a peculiar shaking of the tail so well known to all shepherds, and it may sometimes be seen trying to bite at the part affected. A damp and fœtid patch of wool will usually be found where the maggots are actually at work.

The old maxim " prevention is better than cure " applies to this evil with singular force. If sheep are properly dipped in the early part of summer, they will not be attacked by the Maggot Fly, but it is necessary to remember that non-poisonous or carbolic dips, pitch oil, and things of that kind are absolutely useless against this pest. Cooper's Dip is universally recognized to be not only the best remedy, but the best preventive of the maggot, in existence.

Treatment.—Cut away the wool around, and cleanse the affected parts with a wash made of Cooper's Sheep Dipping Powder and water, made exactly same strength as for dipping—not stronger. If a wound has been made treat as recommended for " wounds."

METRITIS (INFLAMMATION OF THE WOMB).

Two forms of the disease are recognised, simple and septic.—The septic is said to be due to improper management prior to, or at lambing, to exposure during cold, wet seasons, to giving large quantities of rotten turnips, or feeding on coarse innutritious grass. It appears a few hours after parturition. There is dulness, hurried breathing, with straining and discharge of a chocolate-coloured fluid from the uterus, and should the animal live long enough foetid and bloody diarrhœa sets in. Death usually ensues in a few hours.

Treatment is rarely of avail, but similar lines may be carried out to those adopted in cases of simple metritis, with the addition of blood medicines,—perchloride of iron in doses of twenty minims with half a drachm of chlorate of potass being serviceable.

METRITIS (SIMPLE)

usually appears 2 or 3 days after lambing.

Symptoms.—Dulness, frequent change of position, strain-ing, arching of the back, the lips of the vulva being red and swollen. Such cases require prompt attention. Put the animal under shelter, give about two or three ounces of Epsom salts with two drachms of landanum in warm gruel ; inject into the womb an ounce or two of a warm solution of carbolic acid in water 1 to 40 (dissolving the carbolic acid first in glycerine before adding the water), to which a little extract of belladonna has been added. Should the pain continue violent clip the wool off the abdomen and apply mustard over the region of the uterus, and four or five hours after the previous dose give four ounces of linseed oil, with two drachms of laudanum and a drachm and a half of sulphuric ether.

Some have attributed the disease to carelessness on the part of the attendant in not properly cleansing the hands after handling or opening a dead sheep or lamb, but animals which have had no assistance at lambing frequently suffer.

NEPHRITIS IN LAMBS (INFLAMMATION OF THE KIDNEYS).

Lambs suffering from this seldom survive over a fortnight or three weeks. The cause of the disease is somewhat doubtful, but the most probable theory is that which attributes it to weakness or ill-health on the part of the ewe, arising either from constitutional defects or from the animals having been wintered in exposed situations, and on poor innutritious herbage. If that supposition is correct, the means of prevention are obvious.

OPTHALMIA (INFLAMMATION OF THE EYES.)

Sheep are liable to attacks of temporary blindness, most usually arising from exposure to cold and wet, but in other cases due to sudden changes from poor to rich feeding. Symptoms are too well known to need describing. In ordinary cases the disorder rarely lasts over a week or ten days, and treatment is seldom required. Should the animals run any risk of getting into dangerous positions (such as falling into ditches or drains) they should be confined in safer quarters, and be well fed till recovery.

If the bluish film obscuring the sight does not disappear

in a reasonable time, the eye-vein should be punctured, and treatment as below adopted.

The disorder unfortunately sometimes takes an epidemic form in damp localities, and goes through whole flocks, causing serious losses. In outbreaks of this sort the sheep ought to be removed to a high and dry yard; protected from exposure to the glare of the sun, and fed on hay only. Aperient medicines should be administered, and cooling applications, Goulard's extract 1 part, pure rain water 12 parts, frequently applied to the eyes.

PARALYSIS.

This loss of nervous power is, in most cases, only partial, being usually confined to the hind-quarters, and is generally due to long-continued exposure during inclement weather. The victim should be confined under cover, and kept comfortably warm, and have draughts of warm linseed gruel, containing a little powdered gentian and ginger, and a spoonful of brandy or whisky, given twice or thrice a day. If in good condition, it is better policy to slaughter, as in most instances the first loss would be the least.

RICKETS.

A disease of infancy, appearing usually a fortnight or three weeks after birth, caused by cold east winds on certain soils, by in-and-in breeding, and by debility of the dam during pregnancy, the spine and hind-quarters particularly being affected. There is inability to control the movements of the hind limbs, diseased animals frequently reeling and falling down when endeavouring to walk. In this condition they may live some time and even become fairly fat, but should they become incapable of rising, they rapidly waste. The best treatment in such cases is to protect the affected lambs and their mothers from the weather by putting them in a warm dry shed, feed generously, and when the lambs are in sufficiently good condition, kill them. Ewes which have dropped such lambs should not again be bred from. Fewer ewes should be put to each ram, and care should be taken that the condition of both is fairly good when mated, and the feeding of ewes liberal throughout. Change the pasture if at all possible, and give shelter from biting east winds. Oats, as containing the ingredients essential to good bone formation, should be supplied where the pasture is inferior

RUPTURE, OR BROKEN BELLY.

Cases of rupture, or hernia—caused by the weight of the lambs—are occasionally met with amongst ewes when near lambing. The object to be aimed at is keeping the ewe going until after lambing and then feeding her off for the butcher. In some cases keeping them quiet, on small quantities of nourishing food, is all that is necessary. In bad cases some truss or broad band or other support to the abdomen is necessary. A considerable amount of relief will be afforded in very bad cases by getting a piece of strong (but not too heavy) sheet iron, having a few holes pierced along both sides, curved to the shape of the ewe's back, and then passing a piece of canvas beneath the belly, and tying it firmly up to the plate, which is retained in its place by pitch being put on the under side next the wool.

SCAB.

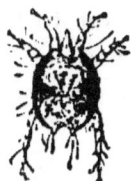

This scourge of flockmasters is caused by the *psoroptes ovis*, a minute parasite just visible to the naked eye. The disease generally shows itself along the sides, extending thence to the back, neck, and rump. The general appearance of infected animals always arouses suspicion in the shepherd. The fleece has a rough broken look. The animals are restless, frequently nibbling at their sides and scratching themselves with their hind feet. In consequence

of this the wool at the elbows is soiled and dirty, and in
horned sheep tufts of wool are frequently seen adhering to
the horns. If the sheep are rubbed gently they manifest
pleasure by smacking their lips. The characteristic lesion
primarily shows itself in the form of whitish or yellowish
pimples which increase in number, and as time goes on
there exudes from these a glutinous fluid, which, combining
with the scurf upon the skin, dries and forms a scab, beneath which the parasites live and multiply, being found in
greatest numbers at the margin of these patches. In extremo
cases, diarrhœa results, or abscesses may appear in various
parts of the body, the animal dying of exhaustion.

The disease is extremely contagious, and its appearance in
the flock is one of the most dreaded incidents in sheep-
farming. The consequent losses are very severe. The animals
fall away in condition and their debility predisposes them to
attacks of other diseases which healthy sheep would resist.

In addition to a very considerable loss in the quantity of
wool its general quality deteriorates, a distinct break in the
fibre occurring as the result of the disease.

The treatment also is expensive, for where an outbreak
occurs it is much better to dip the whole flock; the legal
restrictions are severe, and nobody cares to buy sheep from
an infected flock for a long time afterwards.

Another form of scab known as head scab is due to the
insect *sarcoptes ovis*, and is less serious and more easily
treated. Here the eruption generally appears upon the
muzzle and spreads thence to the face and legs.

With regard to scab it is especially true that prevention is
better than cure. It is a wise precaution to always dip sheep
in Autumn to ensure them against Winter outbreaks which
more frequently occur in those districts where Summer
dipping only is practised; for one dipping can hardly be

expected to preserve the animals from attack for a whole year. All newly purchased sheep should be dipped, and be kept isolated for a time at least.

Treatment.—COOPER'S DIP used according to directions will be found a less expensive and a more effectual remedy than any other. Infected flocks should be strictly isolated. Sheds and yards where such sheep have been housed should be thoroughly cleansed, and these, together with infected pastures and ranges, should be kept unoccupied as long as possible, for it is an established fact that they may retain the infection several months.

SCOUR (SEE DIARRHŒA.)

SHEEP POX.

One of the most destructive and contagious diseases to which sheep are liable, the death rate frequently rising as high as seventy per cent. The duration of the disease is about 28 days. Fortunately, however, it gives British flock-masters little trouble as our sheep are practically exempt from its ravages.

Symptoms.—There is extreme fever, a discharge from the eyes and nose, frequently accompanied by ulceration, salivation, great depression, and disinclination to eat. The body has a most peculiar odour, and fœtid diarrhœa is often present. The specific eruption is best seen in places devoid of wool as in the elbows and the inside of the thighs. There is primarily redness, followed by the appearance of red pimples, the summits of which become surrounded by vesicles whose contents, at first limpid, become ultimately purulent. When an outbreak of this disease occurs, the most economical method of dealing with it is prompt slaughter of the affected animals and those with which they have been in contact, destruction of the carcases by fire and the carrying out of a thorough system of disinfection.

SORE EYES (SEE OPTHALMIA).

If arising from the presence of foreign matter—such as hay-seed—endeavour to remove it, and afterwards apply cooling lotions if the inflammation be severe.

SORE TEATS.

The teats are a frequent source of trouble during wet and frosty weather, more especially if the ewes are short of milk—as the lambs, in their vain endeavours to procure sufficient sustenance, are apt to cut them with their teeth. No more effectual remedy can be employed than a mixture of glycerine and olive oil in equal quantities. Ewes suffering in this manner should be confined in a sheltered place during cold and wet weather. If neglected "inflammation of the udder" usually results.

STURDY, OR GID.

A parasitic disease most common in young sheep up to two years old, due to the lodgment and development in the brain of the cystic form of the *taenia cœnurus cereberalis*, a tapeworm of the dog. Segments of the tapeworm containing mature eggs are expelled from the alimentary canal of the dog, fall on the grass, and are picked up by the sheep when grazing. At first they may cause no inconvenience, but as they develop the brain becomes pressed upon, and nervous symptoms appear. The symptoms vary somewhat according to the locality of the parasite. The animal may appear dull and stupid, one or both ears may be lopped, the pupils of the eyes may be unequal in size. The sheep may persistently turn in one direction, may bore forwards or incline to fall backwards. When the parasite is situated in the the very back of the brain, total paralysis may follow. Animals affected rapidly lose flesh. The sound of running water or the bleating of other sheep seems to possess a special attraction for them. The locality of the parasite can frequently be determined by pressing on the skull, which becomes softened over the spot where the hydatid is lodged. Here the skull may be incised with a trephine (an instrument made for the purpose), and the parasite either removed bodily or its cyst perforated and the fluid allowed to escape. The wound is then closed by the application of a bandage or of tarred tow, and recovery follows if too much brain substance has not been destroyed. As a preventive measure too many dogs should not be permitted on the pasture. All that are kept should receive a dose of vermifuge medicine at intervals of a few months. If animals are in fair condition when first noticed, it is far better to kill them than run the risk of a greater loss.

TAPEWORMS.

The variety of tapeworm that sheep suffer from most frequently is the *Taenia Expansa.* Its segments range from $_2^1$th of an inch at the head to rather over half an inch at the tail. The parasite is found in the intestines of the sheep at all times of the year, and the most common cause of the scourge assuming severe characters is overstocking the pastures, and keeping too many dogs about. The worm grows with great rapidity, having been found 5 yards long in a 4-month old lamb. The egg-bearing segments are expelled in considerable quantities at a time. The immature tapeworm is supposed by some to pass through a phase of existence outside the animal's body before it becomes capable of proper development within the intestines.

Symptoms.—The animals lose condition, become hidebound and bloodless, the appetite is frequently voracious with marked thirst. Diarrhœa sets in, the white oblong segments of the worm are found in the dung, and the animals die from exhaustion.

Treatment.—Withhold food the night before administering medicine, and give no water that morning. Kousso in 1¾ or 2 dram doses may be administered to each lamb, or a dram of oil of male shield fern combined with about 3 ounces of castor oil. This course of treatment is usually satisfactory.

THE TICK.

The *true tick* is fortunately rarely seen in Great Britain, but when once present it is most difficult to get rid of. The female only is parasitic, and burying its head deeply in the skin, clings to its host with stubborn tenacity, and if pulled out leaves an angry looking and painful small wound. The body is very distensible, usually swelling when it is filled with blood into the size of a large horse-bean, which it then closely resembles. When satiated it withdraws its head, and frequently dropping off on the pasture lies there until, becoming again hungry, it attaches itself to another sheep. It may remain apart from the animal for some time. The tick breeds with great rapidity, a large cluster of round eggs issuing from the neck and remaining attached to the body until hatched out.

If neglected, they become a very serious pest, for the quantity of blood they are capable of absorbing is surprising. The flesh of sheep which are attacked by it becomes white, and eventually the animals show signs of extreme debility. The insects burying their heads so deeply, a first dipping may not prove wholly effective, and the operation may require to be repeated not less than a fortnight afterwards. A poisonous dip, remaining in the fleece, and continuing to operate for months after dipping, is the only effective remedy.

TUBERCULOSIS, OR WASTING.

This deadly disorder (the equivalent of consumption in the human being), is fortunately of rare occurrence amongst sheep. It is generally seen among flocks where in-and-in breeding is largely resorted to. The only outward symptoms are a weak and painful cough, failure of appetite, and rapid loss of condition, followed by death. On *post-mortem* examination tubercles are usually discovered in the lungs, liver, and also adhering to the bowels and other viscera. Any attempt at treatment is useless, as the vital organs are fatally undermined by the malady ere any visible signs are given of its existence.

The lambs of any ewes found to have been suffering from this disease should on no account be retained for breeding purposes.

TUMOURS

are frequently seen in sheep, especially in the throat. Many of them are probably of a tubercular nature, and sheep suffering from them should be drafted from the flock. If the tumour is not attached to a bone or to a vital part it may be removed with a knife. In other cases a dressing of tincture of iodine should be applied, and if the tumour forms an abscess and breaks, the wound should be dressed with a little carbolic acid lotion (1 acid to 20 water) and kept open for several days by placing a little wool in it and changing it daily.

WATER ON THE BRAIN (SEE STURDY.)

WOOL BALLS IN LAMBS' STOMACHS.

Heavy losses are sometimes experienced from the accumulation of wool in the stomachs of the lambs. The ordinary symptoms are a complete failure of appetite, accompanied by dulness and giddiness, and death in most cases rapidly ensues,—in many instances, in fact, before anything has been noticed amiss. The lambs of long-woolled ewes are most liable to fall victims, especially if the ewes are in poor condition and short of milk, so that the lambs have to pay

them frequent visits in search of sustenance. All wool
preventing free access to the teats should be clipped away,
in order to lessen the risk of losses in this way.

In other instances the trouble is caused by the presence
of keds or ticks on the bodies of the lambs. The irritation
caused to the latter by these vermin leads them to bite the
itchy parts, and in so doing they are apt to pull out some of
the wool, which is afterwards swallowed by them with their
food. Dipping would prevent trouble arising from this
source.

Whilst the disorder may be said to be almost incurable it
is still possible in some instances to relieve the intestines of
the obstruction by administering frequent doses of castor oil,
and this is the best treatment.

WORMS.

Sheep are rarely troubled by worms except such as already
described, (see Hoose and Tapeworm)—or, at all events, they
seldom show symptoms of it. Their presence gives rise to
inflammation, which may prove fatal. The main symptoms
are a ravenous appetite and unthrifty appearance, and worms
may occasionally be observed in the excrements of the animal.

As treatment a change of feeding should be given, and 2
to 3 drachms of turpentine administered in linseed oil every
third day for three times, on an empty stomach. Salt should
be allowed ad lib., and may be given in the food daily with
½ drachm of sulphate of iron, and 1 drachm sulphur.

WOUNDS.

Probably no domesticated animal suffers so little from
wounds as the sheep; this is on account of the density of
the fleece and its gentle nature. The treatment of simple
wounds is the same as in all other animals. Thorough
bathing with warm water, and afterwards dressing frequently with carbolic lotion (1 acid to 30 water). For maggot
wounds nothing can answer better than this dressing.

THE FROZEN MEAT TRADE.

These modern innovations—steamships and railways—may be said to have "destroyed distance." In a sense the Antipodes are now nearer London than Edinburgh was a century ago.

The improvements effected of late years in the methods of preserving meat—by the process of refrigerating and freezing—have also given a great impulse to the importation of dead meat into Britain from abroad, and the growth of that trade continues steady and enormous.

From a circular recently issued by Messrs. W. Weddel & Co., of London, it appears that in 1880 Australia commenced with a shipment of 400 carcases of sheep. Two years later New Zealand sent us 8,839, the River Plate following, in 1883, with 17,165, and the Falkland Islands, in 1886, with 30,000.

An idea of the rapid strides since made may be obtained by comparing the above "small beginnings" with the shipments of frozen mutton in 1891. During that year

New Zealand contributed	1,896,706
The River Plate	1,073,525
Australia	334,693
Falkland Islands	18,897

Total shipments amounting to 3,323,821 sheep.

In New Zealand there are at present open 17 Refrigerating Works, with a freezing capacity of 3,665,000 carcases per annum, whilst 4 others capable of freezing 500,000 are in the course of construction. In the River Plate there are 4 establishments equivalent to 2,500,000 carcases, and in Australia they have, built and building, a capacity for 1,500,000 carcases annually. The expense of importing this mutton is now reduced to a very small amount. Ship-owners now charge on New Zealand freight 1d. per lb. for mutton,

1½d. per lb. for lamb, and ⅝d. per lb. for beef—these rates covering risk of damage to the meat up to the extent of the freight. River Plate freights vary, but the tendancy is downward. To this may be added storage charges, which have been reduced to ½th of a penny per lb. per month, including cost of landing and delivery, &c., which, with all other "London charges," aggregate, as a rule, to about ⅓rd of a penny per lb. It will thus be seen that 1½d. per lb. now covers the entire cost of transferring this frozen mutton from the Colonial Refrigerator to the hands of the retailer in this country. The average wholesale price of this meat in London may be stated at 3½d. to 4½d. per lb., so that the profits accruing to the rearer abroad from this first part of his business cannot be looked upon as any way excessive— in some cases, indeed, the net return to the breeder has not exceeded 1d. per lb.

That a very large profit is being made by some of those engaged in the meat trade at home is evident when we consider that only a very small fraction of this foreign meat is sold by retail in the British markets under its true name, or at anything approaching the wholesale rates at which it is purchased by the retailers.

Consumers, in fact, seem to be the prey of a host of traders who have not apparently the slightest scruple in disposing of the production of our kinsmen beyond the seas as British meat, and at rates which can only be characterized as utterly exorbitant when compared with its cost.

Were these traders compelled to correctly label their wares a two-fold benefit would result—Home-producers would be relieved from the injustice of imported meat being sold to consumers who might only wish to purchase British, and those consumers whose tastes might lie in the former direction would have the opportunity of buying at more reasonable rates than they can usually do at present.

SHEEP STATISTICS OF THE WORLD.

As an illustration of the vastness of the sheep industry throughout the world it may be mentioned that the number of sheep in the United Kingdom in 1891 was 33,533,988.

In British possessions abroad.

New South Wales	55,986,431
Victoria	12,736,143
South Australia	7,050,544
Western „	2,524,913
Queensland	18,007,234
Tasmania	1,619,256
New Zealand	16,196,048
Fiji Islands	6,838
Total for Australasia	114,127,407
Canada	1,339,695
Cape of Good Hope	13,202,779
Natal	943,117
Ceylon	80,726
Cyprus	213,578
Falkland Islands	676,000
Jamaica	15,044
Malta	14,609
Mauritius	30,000
Newfoundland	42,326
India, West Indies, &c.	uncertain.

SHEEP IN FOREIGN COUNTRIES.

Norway, (1875)	1,686,306
Austria, (1880)	3,841,340
Belguim, (1880)	365,400
Italy, (1882)	6,900,000

Germany, (1883) - - - - - - - -	19,189,715
Russia in Europe, (188) - - : - -	44,465,454
Hungary, (1884) - - - - - - - -	10,594,831
France, (1887) - - - - - - - - -	21,996,731
Holland, (1887) - - - . - - - -	804,300
Sweden, (1889) ' - - - · - - - - -	1,338,195
Denmark, (1888) - - - - - - - -	1,225,196
United States, (1890) - - - - - -	43,431,136
Argentine Republic, (1890) - - - -	70,453,665

IMPORTS AND EXPORTS.

The number of live sheep imported into the United Kingdom in the year 1883 was—

1,116,115 valued at -	- -	£2,518,382
In 1890 358,458 „	- - -	696,312

a decrease of 757,657 in number, and of £1,822,070 in value in the year 1890.

The quantity of fresh mutton imported in 1883 was—

11,824 tons valued at -	-	£696,616
In 1890 82,820 „	„ -	- £3,447,776

an increase of 70,996 tons and of - - £2,751,160 in value of imports in 1890 over those of 1883.

The number of sheep and lambs exported from the United Kingdom in 1890 was 7768, valued at £46,206, or an average of about £5 19s. each.

NAMES OF SHEEP OF DIFFERENT AGES.

The following terms are in vogue in Britain for the various ages of sheep :—

Age.	Male.	Female.
From lambing time till weaned.	tup, or wedder lamb, pur lamb, a heeder.	ewe lamb, a chilver.
From weaning to first shearing or clipping.	wedder teg, tup or wedder hogg or hogget.	ewe teg, ewe hogg, or hogget.
From first to second shearing.	dinmont wedder, shearling ram, or hogg.	gimmer, gimber, (*Lincoln*), threave, 2-tooth shearling ewe.
From second to third shearing.	two-year-old, two-shear ram or wedder.	twinter, two-shear gimmer, *or ewe, if in lamb*, if never put to ram a yeld gimmer, or maiden ewe, if put to ram and no produce a barren gimmer or yeld ewe.

OTHER PROVINCIALISMS EMPLOYED IN NAMING SHEEP.

Cast ewes—Aged ewes drafted and sold from a breeding flock.

Culls, Shotts, or Tails—Sheddings. Inferior sheep selected for rejection.

Cade, or Tiddlin lamb—A pet, one brought up by hand.

Crone—An old broken-mouthed ewe.

Crock, or milled ewe—One that has been crossed with a ram of another breed.

Eild or yeld ewe—A barren ewe.

Guessed ewe—One not seasonably in lamb.

Kebbit ewe—One whose lamb is still-born.

Pallies—Deformed lambs.

Quinter—A sheep from 15 months to 4 years old.

Rig—An imperfectly castrated sheep.

DENTITION OF SHEEP.

The lamb when about a month old possesses eight temporary incisor teeth—usually termed the "milk teeth." The after dentition is considerably affected by the nature of the feeding. When the sheep are on poor keep the centre pair of incisors are "shed" at about one year old, and are replaced by two large and permanent teeth. At about two years old a second pair of large teeth are acquired; at three years old a third pair; and at four years a fourth pair; the animal is then termed "full-mouthed."

When the sheep are liberally fed the first pair of permanent teeth are acquired at about ten months old; the second at eighteen; the third at twenty-seven; and the fourth at about three years. There are however, exceptions to every rule, and the teeth cannot always be relied on in correctly determining the age.

PERIOD OF PREGNANCY.

The duration of pregnancy in the ewe varies slightly; but the average period is about 21 weeks.

AVERAGE MORTALITY.

To state any percentage as a fair average would be mere guess work. With mild seasons and good management the loss is certain to be very much less than that in inclement seasons and in cases where the sheep are not well looked after. Most hill-farmers would consider themselves remarkably fortunate did their annual death-rate over their entire stock not exceed 5 per cent. In many cases however that figure is greatly exceeded. On such farms an average loss of 10 per cent. among the lambs previous to weaning time has been stated to be well within the mark, loss of hoggets between weaning and first clipping 7 per cent., one-shear sheep 6 per cent., two-shear 5 per cent., three or four-shear 4 per cent.

On low-ground farms the losses as a rule are—or at least should be—considerably less. In some known instances not a single death occurred in lamb flocks, numbering about 250, between the time of lambing and weaning, and the average death-rate for the whole flock for the twelve months did not reach 3 per cent.

SHEEP SKINS.

Sheep skins should, if possible, be disposed of immediately after their removal from the carcass, as in a fresh state they are of more value both to buyer and seller than when dried. When, however, they cannot be conveniently got rid of in this manner, they ought to be spread out lengthways, on a stout, rounded, wooden bar, under cover and out of the reach of dogs and other prowlers, until dry. The trotters should not be cut off until the skin has become properly set. When well dried, brush the pelt side thoroughly over with anti-weevil fluid, (procurable from any druggist), to prevent it being destroyed by these insect pests. When the dressing has dried, place the skin carefully aside until sufficient have accumulated to be worth sending off in a body to market.

In packing them for disposal in this manner place them all in one position—the wool side of one skin against the pelt side of another—and secure the bundles firmly by means of rope, or wire, to prevent risk of loss on the journey.

COLONIAL SHEEP FARMING.

The truth of the oft-quoted remark that vast results frequently spring from very small beginnings, was possibly seldom better illustrated than in the rise and progress of the sheep and wool industry in Australasia.

Previous to 1788 no sheep were existant in that part of the world. In that year, however, Botany Bay had the somewhat questionable honour of being selected as the site of a settlement for convicts ; and, with the view of furnishing these unwilling "settlers" and their caretakers with meat and clothing, a consignment of the small hairy sheep of India was imported from Bengal.

In 1797 three Merino rams and five ewes were carried to Australia; and about the year 1801 other three hundred ewes and rams of the merino breed were landed there by the captains of some English whaling ships, who had captured in the South seas, a vessel bound from Spain to Peru with these sheep on board.

These consignments laid the foundation of the sheep industry in Australasia—a business which has within the last twenty years increased to an extent that even the most sanguine could scarcely have anticipated, and which now forms the most durable source of opulence in those important colonies.

Sheep are found to thrive well in almost every part of Australasia, the climate being very favourable—the winters never proving severe, and the heat during summer not being unduly excessive.

The one great drawback with which the Australian flock-masters have to contend is the long-enduring droughts which are periodically experienced, and which not unfrequently sweep off the sheep by hundreds of thousands. In spite of that serious check on the prosperity of the flocks, however, the woolly population of that portion of the globe continues to augment with great rapidity—the increase in numbers since 1873 amounting to no less than 73 per cent.

Until recent times the Colonial sheep-owner had to rely for his profits mainly on the wool-producing power of his flock. The improvements that have lately been made, however, in the methods of preserving meat for an unlimited length of time, by the processes of refrigerating and freezing, give the promise of an increased harvest to the husbandman,—at the expense, "alack-a-day," of us poor mortals of Britishers—and more attention is now being paid to the improvement of the sheep in regard to their mutton-producing properties,

Although, the most of the British breeds are to a certain extent represented in Australasia, the flocks are in great measure—in very many quarters wholly—composed of Merinos; but in districts where the exportation of mutton is making headway, the Leicester-Merino cross is regarded as the most remunerative. The Leicester carries a large quantity of carcase fat, with little fat inside. The Merino has plenty of lean meat and inside fat, and by crossing the two breeds a very profitable mutton sheep is got without depreciating the wool—the cross-bred fleece being found to average about 9 lbs. weight.

New South Wales leads the van in the sheep-rearing industry, possessing about one-half of the aggregate of Australasia. From that district was exported in 1807 the first wool shipped to England from the Colonies. The consignment, which only weighed 245 lbs., was contained in three casks, and shortly after its arrival in London a portion was manufactured, by means of a hand-loom, into a coat for His Majesty King George III.

Extraordinarily high prices are frequently paid for rams by Colonial flock-masters—a "handful of sovereigns" seems to be a mere bagatelle to some of these gentlemen. At the annual Show and Sale under the auspices of the Australian Sheep Breeders Association, at Melbourne, on 23rd August, 1889, a Merino ram from the Scone flock, the property of Messrs. Gibson & Sons, sold for £735. Ten rams from the same gentlemen making an average of £284.

The highest price ever paid for a ram of any breed in Australia was given by the Hon. J. H. Angas, for a Tasmanian-bred Merino ram, which realised the enormous figure of 1,150 guineas.

Severe losses are sometimes experienced by the sheep-owners in various parts of the Colonies owing to the ravages caused by dingoes, or wild dogs; it being necessary in many quarters to fold the sheep at night to protect them from these prowlers.

As we have previously remarked, the Australian flockmaster has been in the past almost wholly dependent on his wool crop for his revenue, and he consequently spares no trouble or expense in preparing it for market.

The sheep are usually washed a few days previous to shearing—pens for containing the animals being erected on the banks of some convenient stream which is, if necessary, dammed up for the purpose, the surplus water passing over the embankment through the medium of wooden spouts. After being soaked in the pool, the animals are passed on to operators standing at the spouts beneath the flow, from which the sheep are confined for a few seconds, until the fleece is thoroughly cleansed from all impurities.

Where a sufficient flow of water is not available for washing in this fashion, and pumping is required, steam-driven gearing has in some instances been erected at great cost. The sheep, after being passed through a tank of cold water, are left for a few hours pretty closely packed together in a 'sweating shed,' furnished with numerous sub-divisions to prevent the sheep crowding so closely together as to run any risk of being smothered. They are then passed through a tank of hot water, usually containing a slight addition of soap, from which the wool is afterwards thoroughly freed by passing the sheep under a spout with cold water. They are then allowed to run free on their pasture until shearing operations are commenced a few days afterwards.

Shearing is wholly performed by "piece-work"—the ordinary rate of payment being 20s. per hundred sheep. As a rule the work is very roughly done, the animals being frequently cut in a manner that would certainly raise the "dander" of even the very best tempered of British flock-masters.

Within the last year or two shearing by machinery has been widely practised. The *sheep-shearing machines* seem destined to prove a boon of incalculable value to the Colonial flockmaster—the work being done much more cleanly and rapidly, even by inexperienced hands, than it could possibly be performed even by the most expert user of the ordinary hand-shears. By its employment the sheep are relieved from the torture of being what has been jokingly termed "skinned alive."

Turning to other parts of the world we find that from North and South America and Africa alike comes the same tale of progress in the sheep industry. Everywhere their numbers are increasing, and more land is being devoted to them. In each of these centres the Merino holds the sway, but in each, also, it is being largely crossed by British breeds. Cattle play a large part in the expansion of a sheep district; they are the pioneers, so to speak, and by eating off the rank grasses give a chance to the finer varieties upon which the sheep mostly thrive.

It might almost be said that the welfare of the human race is largely bound up with the fortunes of this useful quadruped. Certain it is that there are few nooks and crannies throughout this globe of ours, upon which civilization has set its mark, but our four-footed friend is found contributing its quota to the wealth, comfort, and happiness of the community.

INDEX.

M

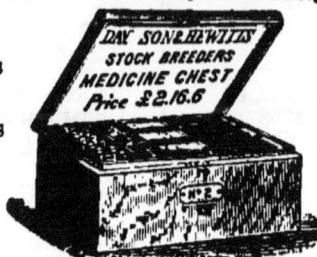

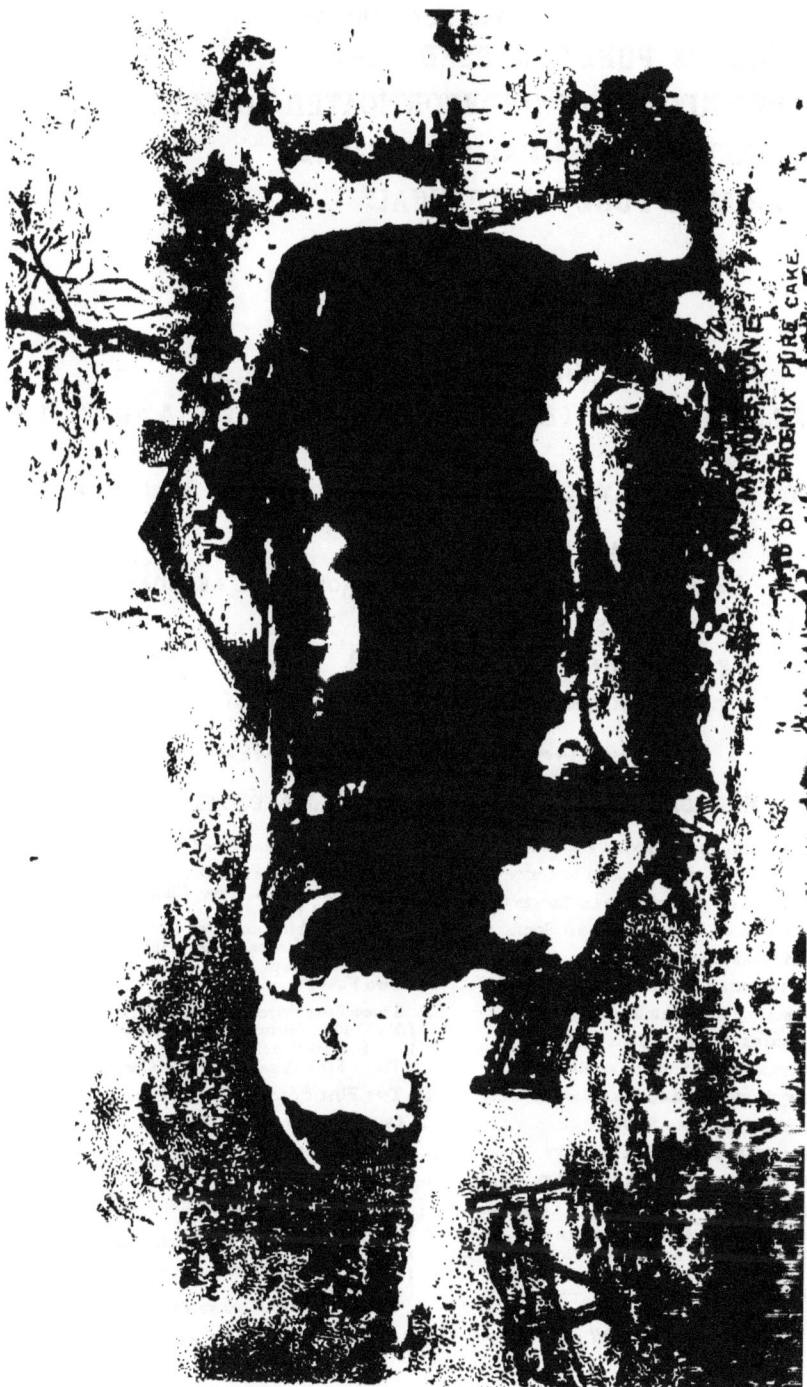

~~~~~~~~~~~~~~~~~~~~~~~~~~~~~~

THE HEREFORD BULL,
MAIDSTONE" (8875), CALVED 20TH APRIL, 1888
BRED BY
H. W. TAYLOR, Esq., Showle Court, Ledbury.

Got by FRANKLIN (6961).

Dam. DUCHESS IV. (vol. xi., p. 302) by TREDEGAR (5077).

g.d., DUCHESS by TWIN (2284).

g.g.d., DUCHESS by ALMA (1144).

g.g.g.d., VICTORIA by PRINCE ALBERT (686).

●●●●●●●●●●●●●●●●●●●●●●●●●●●●●●●●

PRIZES WON BY "MAIDSTONE."

ᴏʏᴀʟ AGRICULTURAL SOCIETY	... Six First Prizes and One Champion Prize (Windsor).
ᴀᴛʜ ᴀɴᴅ Wᴇsᴛ ᴏғ Eɴɢʟᴀɴᴅ SOCIETY	... Three First Prizes and One Champion Prize (Bristol)
ᴇʀᴇFORDSHIRE AGRICULTURAL SOCIETY ... ...{	Five First Prizes, Five Champion Prizes, and O Special Prize.
HROPSHIRE AND WEST MIDLAND SOCIETY	... Two First Prizes and Two Champion Prizes.
LOUCESTERSHIRE AGRICULTURAL SOCIETY ... ...{	Four First Prizes, One Champion Prize, and O Special Cup.
ᴼORCESTERSHIRE AGRICULTURAL SOCIETY	... Two First Prizes.
LANORGANSHIRE AGRICULTURAL SOCIETY	Three First Prizes and Three Champion Prizes.
xFORDSHIRE AGRICULTURAL SOCIETY .. ..{	Two First Prizes, One Champion Prize, and O Special Prize.
BERGAVENNY AGRICULTURAL SOCIETY	Three First Prizes and Three Champion Prizes.
UDLOW AGRICULTURAL SOCIETY	Two First Prizes and Two Champion Prizes.
SSEX AGRICULTURAL SOCIETY	One First Prize.
HERBORNE AGRICULTURAL SOCIETY	One First Prize.
EOMINSTER AGRICULTURAL SOCIETY	One First Prize.
ᴏʏᴀʟ COUNTIES AGRICULTURAL SOCIETY	One First Prize and One Champion Prize.
ᴏʏᴀʟ LIVERPOOL & MANCHESTER AGRICULTURAL } SOCIETY	One First Prize and One Champion Prize.
ᴏʏᴀʟ DUBLIN SOCIETY .. ..{	First Prize, Chaloner Plate, and Gibbs Challenge C in 1885. First Prize and Chaloner Plate in 1887.

As well as numerous other valuable and important prizes.

THE FRIEND

OF

THE FARMER.

—⊢→⇒⊛⊂←⊢—

THE BEST PENNY SPENT ON THE FARM IS IN DIPPING.

—⊢→⇒⊛⊱←⊢—

THE BEST DIP IS

COOPERS DIPPING POWDER.

—⊢→⇒⊛⊂←⊢—

EVERY SHILLING

SPENT ON THIS DIP

BRINGS BACK TEN.

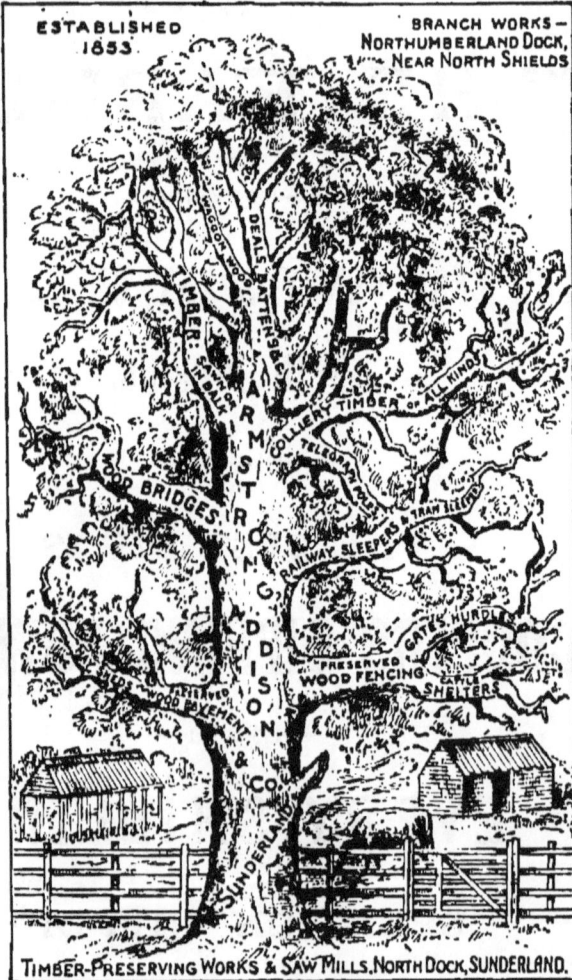

ESTD. 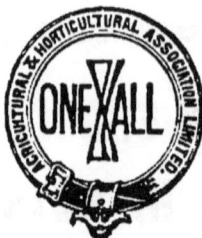 1867.

AGRICULTURAL & HORTICULTURAL ASSOCIATION, LIMITED.

A purely mutual society of 3000 Landowners and Farmers. The pioneer society for the co-operative supply of Farm Requisites of guaranteed quality at wholesale prices. Supplies its members and the public with goods produced and imported by the Association.

COMPLETE MANURES,
RELIABLE SEEDS,
PURE OIL-CAKES,

SPECIAL CAKES for milk production, for speedy fatting, and for young stock.

IMPLEMENTS AND MACHINERY.

Details and Catalogues post free on application.

Edwd. Owen Greening

3, Agar St., Strand, W.C., and Deptford, S.E.

Managing Director.

AGRICULTURAL & HORTICULTURAL ASSOCIATION, LIMITED,

Creek Rd., Deptford, S.E., and 3, Agar St., Strand, W.C.

FEEDING CAKE, No. 2.

A Special Food for Lambs, Sheep, and Store Cattle generally.

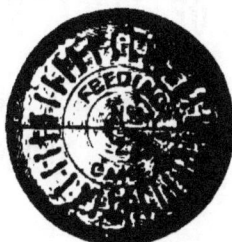

GUARANTEED ANALYSIS:—

Oil 6 to 7 per cent; Albuminoids 17 to 19 per cent; Mucilage, Sugar, &c., 51 to 53 per cent.

STORE CAKE No. 4.

A cheaper Cake for Store Cattle. Made of pure material.

GUARANTEED ANALYSIS:—

Oil 4 to 5 per cent; Albuminoids 20 to 22 per cent; Mucilage, Sugar, &c., 49 to 52 per cent.

Delivered free on rails, at either London, Liverpool, Bristol, Hull, or Southampton.

Full Particulars and present Prices on application to

Edw. Owen Greening.

3, Agar St., Strand, W.C., and Deptford, S.E.

Managing Director.

THE STRUCTURE

OF THE

WOOL FIBRE,

IN ITS RELATION TO THE

USE OF WOOL FOR TECHNICAL PURPOSES;

Illustrated with numerous Engravings and Coloured Plates.

BY

F. H. BOWMAN, D.Sc., F.R.S.E., F.L.S.,

Fellow of the Chemical Society; Fellow of the Institute of Chemistry;
Fellow of the Royal Microscopical Society; Member of the Society
of Arts and Manufactures; Fellow of the Society of Chemical
Industry; Vice-President of the Society of Dyers and
Colourists; Straton Prizeman and Gold Medallist
in Technology, University of Edinburgh.

SECOND EDITION.

MANCHESTER :

PALMER AND HOWE, 73, 75, & 77, PRINCESS STREET,
LONDON : SIMPKIN, MARSHALL, & Co.,
PHILADELPHIA : HENRY CAREY BAIRD & Co.

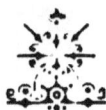

ARTHUR FINN,

Westbroke,

LYDD, Kent.

PURE

ROMNEY MARSH SHEEP.

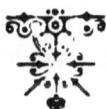

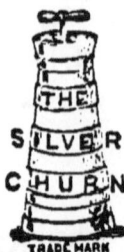

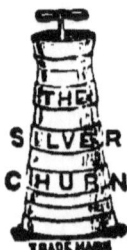

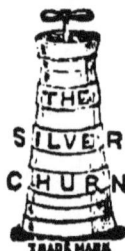

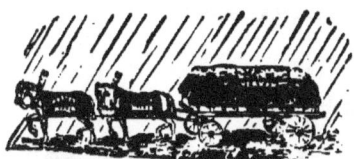

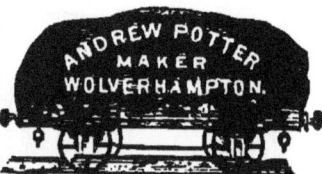

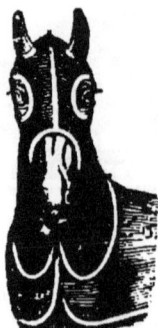

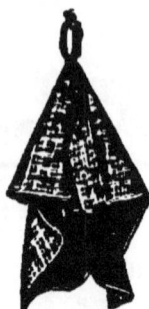

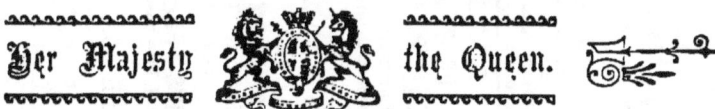

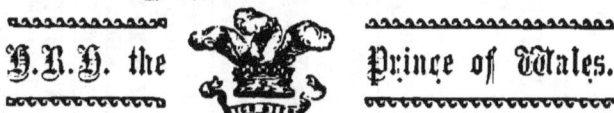

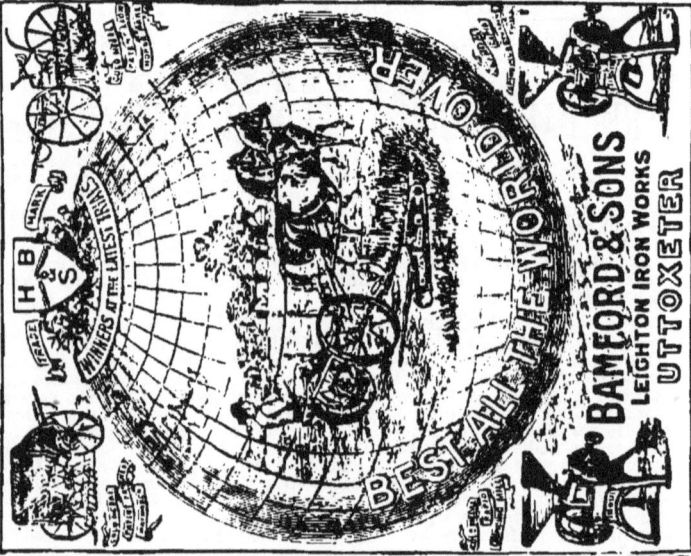

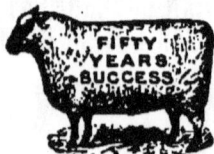

CLASS.	PRIZES.	EXHIBITOR'S NAME & ADDRESS.
HAMPSHIRE DOWN.		
Two-Shear Ram	SECOND	F. R. Moore, Littlecott, Upavon, Marlborough.
Shearling Ram	FIRST	J. Barton, Hackwood Farm, Basingstoke.
Pen of 3 Ram Lambs	SECOND	" " "
SUFFOLK.		
Two-Shear Ram	FIRST	Marquis of Bristol, Ickworth Park, Bury-St.-Edmunds.
"	SECOND	T. L. Roberson & W. Gough, Hengrave, Bury-St.-Edmunds.
"	THIRD	Marquis of Bristol.
Shearling Ram "	SECOND	
" "	THIRD	T. L. Roberson & W. Gough.
Pen of 3 Ram Lambs	FIRST	Marquis of Bristol.
Pen of 3 Shearling Ewes ...	FIRST	J. Smith, Thorpe Hall, Hasketon, Woodbridge, Suffolk.
" " " ...	SECOND	T. L. Roberson & W. Gough.
" " " ...	THIRD	Marquis of Bristol.
WENSLEYDALE.		
Two-Shear Ram	FIRST	J. O. Trotter, Holtby Grange, Bedale.
" "	SECOND	J. Hough, Mudd Fields, Bedale.
Shearling Ram	FIRST	" " "
" "	SECOND	
" "	THIRD	J. O. Trotter.
Pen of 3 Ram Lambs	FIRST	J. Hough.
Pen of 3 Shearling Ewes ...	FIRST	" "
" " " ...	SECOND	" "
BORDER LEICESTER.		
Ram...	FIRST	Rt. Hon. A. J. Balfour, M.P., Whittinghame, Prestonkirk, Haddingtonshire
"	THIRD	" " "
Shearling Ram	FIRST	" " "
Pen of 3 Shearling Ewes ...	FIRST	" " "
" " " ...	SECOND	" " "
CHEVIOT.		
Ram...	FIRST	Jacob Robson, Byrness, Otterburn, Northumberland.
"	SECOND	John Robson, Newton, Bellingham.
Shearling Ram	FIRST	" "
" "	SECOND	Jacob Robson.
Pen of 3 Shearling Ewes ...	FIRST	John Robson.
" " " ...	SECOND	Jacob Robson.
LONK.		
Ram...	SECOND	J. Blackburn, Holling Hall, Trawden, Lancs.
HERDWICK.		
Ram...	SECOND	J. C. Bowstead, Chapel Hill, Mardale, Penrith.
Shearling Ram	FIRST	" " "

THE SALE OF

COOPER'S DIP

ADVANCES BY LEAPS AND BOUNDS.

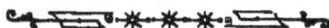

OFFICIAL CERTIFICATE.

41, Coleman Street, London, E.C.,

2nd February, 1892.

We have examined the books of Messrs. Wm. Cooper & Nephews, of Berkhamsted, and we certify that the sales of their Sheep Dipping Powder for the year ended 31st December, 1891, are In excess of those for the previous year by 1,140,170 Packets, or 890 tons 15 cwt. 17 lbs.

TURQUAND, YOUNGS, WEISE, BISHOP, & CLARKE,

Accountants.

Farmers may be presumed to know what is best for their flocks.

THIS IS THEIR VERDICT.

www.ingramcontent.com/pod-product-compliance
Lightning Source LLC
Chambersburg PA
CBHW021941220326
41599CB00013BA/1482